LIFE AT A DISTANCE

EXPERTISE

**CULTURES AND
TECHNOLOGIES
OF KNOWLEDGE**

EDITED BY DOMINIC BOYER

A list of titles in this series is available at cornellpress.cornell.edu.

LIFE AT A DISTANCE

Medicine and Nationalism
in India's Pan-African
e-Network

Vincent Duclos

CORNELL UNIVERSITY PRESS   **ITHACA AND LONDON**

First published 2025 by Cornell University Press

Librarians: A CIP catalog record for this book is available from the Library of Congress.

ISBN 9781501782053 (hardcover)
ISBN 9781501782060 (paperback)
ISBN 9781501782077 (epub)
ISBN 9781501782084 (pdf)

Pour Émile et Béatrice

Contents

Acknowledgments

This book bears the mark of so many conversations and encounters. Research presented in the book was conducted over one decade, and so many people generously shared their time, their knowledge, and their craft with me along the way. I first want to thank the many actors of the Pan-African e-Network (PAN) who introduced me to their work and provided me with advice and orientation. PAN always was the source of great pride and ambition, which made it, at times, a sensitive object of investigation. Nevertheless, many telemedicine pioneers and supporters of the network have kindly opened their doors to me. In India, this includes the late president of India Abdul Kalam as well as Profs. Krishnan Ganapathy, S. K. Mishra, and Arun Tiwari, among many others. I am also indebted to former TCIL managers for facilitating this research to the extent they deemed possible. In Dakar, I want to thank the telemedicine team at CHNU Fann, including Prof. Bara Diop, Marieme Ndoye, Jean-Louis Manga, Sada Dia, and Dr. Mohamed Leye, for welcoming this research with great generosity. Both in India and on the African continent, I am extremely grateful to the numerous telemedicine engineers who have introduced me to their work. I have spent a significant amount of time with engineers, and I still cherish friendships with some of them. The engineers made the Pan-African e-Network possible, and this book is largely dedicated to them. This being said, I bear full responsibility for the materials presented in this manuscript, for any inaccuracy it might contain, and for the analysis I propose.

During the decade researching and writing this book, I have had the privilege to occupy different academic positions and work with great colleagues. In the department of anthropology at the Université de Montréal, I met mentors and friends who have accompanied and nourished this research at many different stages. This includes Bernard Bernier, Suzanne Beth, Erik Bordeleau, Kim Turcot DiFruscia, Sylvie Fortin, Karine Gagné, Léa Kalaora, Chowra Makaremi, Anne Lardeux, and Bob White. In the Department of Social Studies of Medicine at McGill University, I have benefited from conversations and support from Tobias Rees, George Weisz, Allan Young, and Nick King. I am also thankful to Madhu Pai for the support provided by McGill's Global Health Program. Between 2017 and 2020, I taught and did research at Drexel University, with a joint appointment in the Center for STS and the Department of Global Studies and Modern Languages. At Drexel, I have received great support and mentorship from Susan Bell, Mary Ebeling, Kelly Joyce, Ali Kenner, Rogelio Miñana, Nada Matta, Gwen

Ottinger, Mimi Scheller, and Chloe Silverman, among others. The conversations I had with Drexel colleagues were instrumental in shaping the key argument of the book. I now have the great privilege to work at the Université du Québec à Montréal (UQAM), a major French-language public university with a unique history of progressive politics and a model of bottom-up governance that challenges the corporatization of higher education. It is my hope that some of UQAM's spirit of solidarity and resistance has found its way into this book. I am very thankful to all of my colleagues at the Département de communication sociale et publique, and particularly to the department chair Chantal Aurousseau, for making me feel at home when I moved into a new position in the midst of a global pandemic.

In many different ways, this book was inspired by numerous colleagues and friends including Vincanne Adams, Marine Al Dahdah, Dörte Bemme, Cal Biruk, Victor Braitberg, Charlotte Brives, Carlo Caduff, Pierre-Marie David, Janice Graham, Frédéric Keck, Janina Kehr, Claudia Lang, Catherine Larouche, SoYeon Leem, Céline Lefève, Caroline Meier zu Biesen, Alex Nading, Canay Ozden-Schilling, Tom Ozden-Schilling, Johannes Quack, Mathieu Quet, Emilia Sanabria, Nick Shapiro, Alice Street, and Oumy Thiongane. For many years, I have been a lucky member of Translating Vitalities, a unique and vibrant community of artists, scholars, and health practitioners. Collective thinking and experiments with Sue Cochrane, Judith Farquhar, Stacey Langwick, William Mazzarella, Carla Nappi, Barry Saunders, Volker Scheid, and Clare Twomey, among other members of the collective, were hugely influential in developing my thinking about some of the topics found in this book.

Over the years, I was also able to share some of the key arguments of this book with great audiences by way of invited lectures, a writing group, workshops, conference talks, or journal articles. For invitations and discussions, I am particularly grateful to Dan Banik, Sandra Bärnreuther, Marian Burchardt, Sandra Caulkins, Susan Erickson, Abou Farman, Jean-Paul Gaudillière, Jeremy A. Greene, Kenneth King, Julie Livingston, Celia Lowe, Tom Neumark, Robert Peckham, Richard Rottenburg, Smriti Sharma, Katerini Storeng, and Meera Venkatachalam. I also want to thank Tomás Sánchez Criado, Vincent Laliberté, Jean-Michel Landry, Ramah McKay, Pierre Minn, Gwen Ottinger, Laura Risk, Noémi Tousignant, and two anonymous reviewers for their careful reading and insightful comments on draft chapters of the manuscript. The book has also benefited from collaborations on related digital health research in West Africa with colleagues and graduate students including Sylvain Landry Faye, Moubassira Kagoné, Ourohiré Millogo, Tidiane Ndoye, Hamidou Sanou, N. Hélène Sawadogo, Ali Sié, Georgette Sow, Martine Eva Tine, and Maurice Yé. At Cornell University Press and Amnet, I want to thank Dominic Boyer, Jennifer Crane, Jim Lance, Alfredo Gutierrez Rios, Susan P. Specter, and Bethany Wasik for their invaluable support every step of the way.

The research leading to this book has greatly benefited from a Joseph-Armand Bombardier CGS Doctoral Scholarship, awarded by the Social Sciences and Humanities Research Council of Canada (SSHRC), and a Fernand Braudel Postdoctoral Fellowship from the Collège d'études mondiales (Paris). Segments of the introduction and of chapter 4 were previously published as "The Empire of Speculation," *Biosocieties* 16 (2021): 289–311. Portions of chapter 5 were previously published as "Map and Territory: An Ethnographic Study of the Low Utilization of a Global eHealth Network," *Journal of Information Technology* 31, no. 4 (2016): 334–46.

Over the past decade or so, some friends and mentors have provided me with constant, invaluable encouragement at both personal and intellectual levels. I want to express particular gratitude for the relationships developed with Gilles Bibeau, Judith Farquhar, and Miriam Ticktin, all of whom have been formidable friends and supporters of this project at various stages. Vinh-Kim Nguyen was a thoughtful supervisor and mentor during my years as a graduate student and beyond. I could not have asked for better accompaniment. Over the years, I was privileged to belong to a group of closely knit friends, most nonacademic, most brilliant, uncertain what this manuscript is about, and considerate enough not to inquire about its status. They know who they are. This book would not have been possible without the unwavering support of my parents and of my brother over the years and in all spheres of life. I can't thank them enough. Beyond all, I dedicate this book to Andrée-Anne for her clever, joyful, caring companionship that makes everyday life feel like home wherever we are.

Abbreviations

AIIMS	All India Institute of Medical Sciences
APPLE	Ariane Passenger PayLoad Experiment
ATNF	Apollo Telemedicine Networking Foundation
AUC	African Union Commission
BJP	Bharatiya Janata Party
CHNU	Centre hospitalier national universitaire (National University Hospital)
CME	Continuing Medical Education
DTCS	Department of Thoracic and Cardiovascular Surgery
GDP	Gross Domestic Product
IAFS	India–Africa Forum Summit
INCOSPAR	Indian National Committee for Space Research
INSAT	Indian National Satellite System
IPLC	International Private Leased Circuit
ISRO	Indian Space Research Organisation
ISU	International Space University
ITEC	Indian Technical and Economic Cooperation
MPI	Moon Probe Impact
NASA	National Aeronautics and Space Administration
NDM-1	New Delhi metallo-beta-lactamase 1
NIIT	National Institute of Information Technology
PAN	Pan-African e-Network Project
RASCOM	Regional African Satellite Communication Organization
SAARC	South Asian Association for Regional Cooperation
SEA-ME-WE 4	South East Asia–Middle East–Western Europe 4
SGPGIMS	Sanjay Gandhi Postgraduate Institute of Medical Sciences
SITE	Satellite Instructional Television Experiment
TCIL	Telecommunications Consultants India Ltd.
UPS	Uninterruptible Power Supply
VSAT	Very Small Aperture Terminal
WHO	World Health Organization

LIFE AT A DISTANCE

Introduction

It was 1:45 p.m. in Chennai, in the south of India. Like every day, Ashoka[1] fiddled with the production switcher, making sure that the audio and video quality were good enough. He went back and forth between the control room and the studio. He adjusted the camera. He returned to his workstation to reply to a colleague writing from the Institut Médical de Madagascar in Antananarivo. Then to another one in Dakar, Senegal. Everything was set. The PowerPoint presentation was ready. The communication was stable. We just had to wait now.

It was an afternoon like any other in the large, air-conditioned premises of Apollo Hospital in Chennai. Over the past two years, thousands of continuing medical education (CME) sessions had been broadcast as part of the Pan-African e-Network Project. Among these, a significant percentage was given from this flagship Indian corporate hospital. This was on top of the medical teleconsultations, which were much more common in Apollo than in most other Indian hospitals connected to the network. On days when both CME sessions and teleconsultations took place, things could get busy. Ashoka had to ensure that the communication was good, that the diagnostic images were all properly scanned, that doctors showed up on time, and that medical records were fully uploaded into the network's electronic medical system. Days with no session at all were quieter. We listened to music. We visited the neighboring offices of the Apollo Telemedicine Networking Foundation. We chatted with colleagues dispatched across India and the African continent. We talked about everything and nothing. We watched time pass by.

Today, Ashoka was visibly satisfied. He pointed to the screen: "You see today, good attendance." Out of the thirty hospitals, spread over as many countries, in which Dr. Aggarwal's talk was about to be broadcast, some boasted a considerable audience. In a few minutes, the cardiologist would be presenting a talk on the management of coronary heart disease. He would be speaking for half an hour. Then there might be some questions. Dr. Aggarwal would be sitting alone behind a table, looking at a camera but also at the screen in front of him with images of residents and doctors sitting calmly thousands of miles away, listening and taking notes. Others would talk, get busy, and argue without paying attention to the talk. But especially, despite this being a good day, he'd be staring at images of empty chairs.

Ashoka remained alert. He kept monitoring the network, making sure it was holding up and that there weren't any bugs. Ashoka then turned to me: "You know, Mr. Vincent, we are taking care of the world. We are making their lives better."

~~~

In September 2004, the president of India, Dr. Abdul Kalam, proposed to connect Africa and India through a network infrastructure that would provide telemedicine and tele-education services. Five years later, on February 26, 2009, the Pan-African e-Network Project, or PAN, was launched. *Life at a Distance* tells the story of PAN and specifically of its global telemedicine—also referred to as *digital health* or *digital medicine*—network.[2] PAN was an ambitious project. Implemented by Telecommunications India Limited (TCIL), a public Indian company very active in Africa, it was the largest telemedicine project on the African continent (Dihel and Goswami 2016, 66). A major investment funded entirely by the Indian government, PAN was also the largest single development or global health project undertaken by India abroad.[3] The network operated continually between 2009 and 2017, and a new version is apparently being deployed at the moment of writing.[4] PAN's telemedicine network connected twelve tertiary-care hospitals in India with over thirty hospitals located in as many African countries. It delivered two kinds of medical services: teleconsultations and continuing medical education. Put simply, PAN aimed to care for patients at a distance. PAN was an infrastructure in the basic sense of a built material form that allows for the possibility of exchange over space (Larkin 2013, 328). It accelerated the flows of capital, expertise, and technology between India and Africa. Beyond its technical or medical operations, however, PAN also existed as a state of desire. *Life at a Distance* attends to the speculative logic of PAN as a flagship South-South capitalism project.[5] It examines how PAN conjured certain futures for the Indian nation and the world beyond familiar Western-centric scripts.

This book makes two distinct yet related arguments. First, the book suggests that, as a "shining example of South-South cooperation" (the slogan of the project), PAN challenged Western hegemony and speculated on "the South" as an emergent economic, medical, political, and technological formation. PAN desta-bilized assumptions, dominant in global health spheres, about the circulation of technology and medicine along North-South geopolitical lines. In spite of some examples of South-South assistance, the history of global health—and indeed of global capital—remains mainly concerned with flows of goods, services, and strat-egies along North-South pathways (Packard 2016). This state of affairs, however, is changing rapidly as emerging powers such as China and India are becoming key stakeholders in sub-Saharan Africa. PAN was funded by the Indian state to sup-port Indian hospitals as they sought to make inroads into African health care mar-kets. It aimed to counter China's growing presence in the medical and technology sectors in Africa. Beyond mere economic interests, however, PAN performed a moral defense of an Indian brand of global capitalism. PAN's stakeholders had no time for the Euro-American language of humanitarian aid or assistance. Affective investments in PAN were shaped by different world-historical trajectories (Biehl and Locke 2017, 28).

Life at a Distance retraces these trajectories as it examines the history of trade and cooperation between Africa and India. It explores the lasting power of the past, including of nostalgic accounts of characters such as Jawaharlal Nehru or events like the Bandung Conference, in shaping the imagination of future South-South relations. Although PAN had little in common with the hopes for collective emancipation often associated with an event like Bandung, it certainly shared a sentiment that the Global North is no longer the primary agentive force or the center of gravity of the world. As chapter 1 suggests, however, PAN materialized a shift in the philosophy of cooperation between India and Africa, which is best encapsulated by the phrase of former Indian prime minister Manmohan Singh: "Cooperation is trade, not aid." A public-private partnership, PAN staged a corpo-rate version of the Indian state, which invests heavily to support Indian hospitals as they seek to build a presence in African health care markets. PAN facilitated the outsourcing of medical expertise and established relations between patients, doctors, and institutions. *Life at a Distance* can thus be read as an ethnography of dream-making and its economic logic (Bear, Birla, and Puri 2015, 389). However, although the network did produce economic value, its affective drive operated beyond mere commercial logic. In PAN, market expansion was animated by a desire for national grandeur and revival. PAN was at once a flagship project and an aesthetic object through which the uniqueness of the Indian nation was marketed and nationhood produced. It was a medium for the Indian nation to perform itself as an aspirant caregiver and power. As such, PAN appears as a strategic location to critically explore how nationalist convulsions energize global health and indeed global capitalism. It raises the questions: How does a large network of medical enclaves in Africa contribute to the imagination of India? How does the nation extend and shape itself, as a political and spatial formation, by intervening in the lives of other, remote peoples?

In a second line of argument, *Life at a Distance* suggests that, as it speculated about and accelerated transnational flows between Indian and African hospitals, the Pan-African e-Network created connected enclosures: networked but enclaved medical spaces carved out of fragile, unstable connections. The book describes the labor, technical routines, and material infrastructures that crafted and sustained these medical spaces. The launch of PAN involved extending a transnational network infrastructure composed of a fiber-optic network, undersea cables, and satellite connectivity as well as various computer and medical equipment. *Life at a Distance* documents how PAN brought together designers, medical practitioners, politicians, medical and technological corporations, and hospital and project managers. Challenging the promise of digital networks to deterritorialize physical space, this book shows the kind of mediation work that exists between clinical worlds in Africa and India. Some patients get access to treatment while others don't. Doctors get frustrated with the broken promises of reciprocity. Medical work in PAN was constrained by material, organizational, and spatial enclosures. It was contingent on the network as physical, aesthetic, and political form: on affordances, patterns, and topologies that shaped the way human life was made visible and intervened upon at a distance. *Life at a Distance* offers a glimpse into emergent medical forms in times where "human bodies, networks, and place all propagate into one other, making it more difficult to say what is life and what is not life" (TallBear 2011). At the core of the story lies the complex interplay of inside and outside, expansion and containment, speculation about the future, and the hard-edged enclosures of the present—in the clinic and beyond.[6]

Enclosures

Omar was a four-year-old Senegalese boy who was hospitalized at the Centre Hospitalier Universitaire de Fann (CHNU Fann) in Dakar. Omar suffered from a chronic heart condition, and the medical team at Fann believed that he needed a pacemaker. However, having never seen a similar case, the cardiologists at Fann were unsure about the sort of pacemaker they should install in such a young child. Pediatric cardiology was relatively new at Fann hospital. Until recently, a case like this one would have been transferred abroad. After discussing Omar's case during a staff meeting, the medical team decided to ask their Indian colleagues for advice. They would connect to PAN. The next day, a teleconsultation took place between Omar's doctor, Dr. Leye, and Dr. Kumar, a pediatric cardiologist from Fortis Hospital in Delhi. During the session, Dr. Kumar and Dr. Leye reviewed Omar's medical record, scrolling through and commenting on scan images. Dr. Kumar insisted that Omar needed to have the pacemaker installed as soon as possible. Then, for almost an hour, he guided Dr. Leye through the surgical procedure. One week later, Omar underwent a successful surgery. Months later, Dr. Leye still spoke of the clinical encounter with a sense of satisfaction. For their part, Omar and his parents were never aware that a teleconsultation took place before he underwent surgery.

Teleconsultations in PAN covered a dozen medical specialties, with radiology, neurology, and pediatric care being among the most common. Teleconsultations were provided free of charge to African hospitals, although participating Indian hospitals were subsidized by TCIL—and, ultimately, the Ministry of External Affairs—to provide them. Teleconsultations took place in studios equipped for this purpose with communication and medical devices. They consisted of videoconference sessions between Indian specialists and their African colleagues in which they discussed patient cases, clinical impressions, probable diagnoses, and advisable treatments. Usually requested by medical teams in participating African hospitals to address challenging patient cases, teleconsultations could be used to obtain a second opinion when a diagnosis was uncertain. They could also provide support in the therapeutic management of patients and in assisting doctors who were inexperienced with performing certain procedures.[7] In some participating African hospitals, such as CHNU Fann, teleconsultations with Indian medical specialists became a key part of the treating team's "diagnostic ritual."[8] Dr. Ndiaye, a neurologist at CHNU Fann hospital, summed up the impact of teleconsultations in this way: "The network broadens our vision. It opens it up to all sorts of possibilities in terms of diagnosis and therapy."[9]

At first glance, Dr. Ndiaye might seem to confirm one of the main expectations associated with PAN, and indeed with telemedicine—namely, that digital technologies can deterritorialize the circulation of and access to medical expertise and care.[10] Ethnographic inquiry into PAN, however, complicates this promise by revealing how conflicted, contradictory medical spaces are carved out and sustained. *Life at a Distance* makes visible the infrastructural history, materialities, and labor practices involved in mediating relations between medical worlds in Africa and India. Nonclinical labor and spaces were the conditions of possibility for medicine in PAN. The Pan-African e-Network was made of one inland fiberoptic cable network within India, two submarine communications cable systems— namely SEA-ME-WE 4 and ATLANTIS-II—connecting India with Africa, and satellite technology. To connect its African sites, PAN used the RASCOM-QAF1 satellite. Launched into orbit in 2007, a few months before PAN began its activities, RASCOM-QAF1 was the first satellite entirely dedicated to the African continent. RASCOM-QAF1, later replaced by RASCOM-QAF1R, aimed to provide affordable bandwidth and support regional autonomy and cooperation. It was a Pan-African response to the Western domination of the satellite market. PAN's network infrastructure was thus deeply entrenched within historical struggles, territorialities, and regional imaginaries. Its everyday operations also relied on the labor of dozens of engineers dispatched across India and the African continent. Two engineers worked full-time on the project at all participating hospitals. Others worked in the network's data centers. Hired by TCIL, engineers executed a range of tasks such as scheduling teleconsultations, managing bandwidth, and perfecting image and sound quality. They administered medical data and thus played a key role in patient care. The infrastructure of PAN, then, was sustained by repetitive, routine work performed behind the scenes.

In conversation with the work of theorists who have engaged with the many entanglements of the human and the machine, the semiotic and the material, *Life at a Distance* proposes an ecological, relational understanding of telemedicine.[11] PAN emerged *in practice* through relations with activities, people, and other existing structures.[12] For example, participating doctors often had to adapt courses of treatment according to the local availability of diagnostic testing or medicines. Failing connectivity or language barriers could come with concrete health consequences. And patients diagnosed remotely oftentimes could not afford treatment or to travel abroad for medical care—reinforcing already existing patterns of exclusion.

Take the case of Aasiya, discussed in greater detail in chapter 3.[13] At the time of the teleconsultation via PAN, Aasiya was hospitalized at the Bosaso General Hospital, a public hospital in Northern Somalia. A woman in her thirties, Aasiya was experiencing symptoms of generalized itching, abdominal pain, dark urine, and fever. The teleconsultation involved her attending physician and a gastroenterologist from Apollo Hospital in Chennai. About fifteen minutes into the discussion, the doctors agreed on a probable diagnosis. However, the Indian gastroenterologist insisted that an abdominal CT scan was required before any surgical procedure was performed. This was not an option, explained Aasiya's attending physician, because the hospital did not have a CT scanner. His Indian colleague then inquired about the possibility of Aasiya traveling to India for treatment. Aasiya explained that she could not afford to pay for treatment abroad. Both physicians then agreed to nevertheless go ahead with the surgery, for lack of better options. A case like Aasiya's shows how telemedicine generates new contexts of uncertainty and improvisation.[14] As chapter 3 will suggest, however, uncertainty was not evenly distributed in PAN: by design, certain relations were enabled while others were not.

The Pan-African e-Network was connecting hospitals spread over thirty countries. It integrated private and public hospitals in metropolises and small towns while operating in multiple languages and time zones and highly variable condi-

tions. The network sutured discrepant places as nodes within larger infrastructures of informational and medical flows (Simone 2018, 127). To tame the difference between sites, TCIL officers liked to insist that the network was designed
as a "turnkey solution."[15] A turnkey approach relied on a series of enclosures.
First, there were technological enclosures. PAN was designed to be operational
in a wide range of conditions—for instance, in hospitals with unstable power
supplies, poor telecommunication facilities, or a shortage of skilled labor. To do
so, it came with an entire system of technical support: a "portability kit" including a UPS device as well as medical and computer equipment.[16] The network
also comprised an electronic medical record system to facilitate the standardized
circulation of patient data. The kit resembled the "kit system" described by Peter
Redfield (2013) in *Life in Crisis*, his ethnography of Doctors without Borders.
The kit is a *global*, mobile system, not at all fluid in terms of local appropriation.
But while the Doctors without Borders' kit was designed as a means for crisis
response, PAN's was designed for stable, lasting network operability.

Enclosures were also spatial and topological. For example, in the vast majority
of the participating hospitals I have visited, PAN's studios were physically remote
from the hospital wards. They were insulated, air-conditioned spaces connected
to hospitals yet isolated from their day-to-day operations. Studios would sometimes be located in a separate building or at the end of a hallway. TCIL's turnkey
approach was also embedded in the topology of the network itself.

PAN connected participating sites using a star topology. Put simply, on a star
network all communications need to be channeled through a hub. This stands
in contrast to a mesh network in which nodes can communicate with each other
without going through the hub. The star topology, project designers explained
to me, prevented unsolicited connection to the network. As I explain in chapter
3, while the star topology enabled a centralized expansion in which TCIL could
control transnational flows, it also rigidified the network and compromised possibilities for improvisation.

The production and distribution of expertise in PAN were thus contingent
on enclosures that sheltered the network from the singularity of connected sites
and territories. Network connectivity in PAN imposed order on space, reified
distinctions among peoples and places, and shaped the possibilities to know,
imagine, and intervene upon life at a distance. As such, PAN was illustrative of
a contradiction driving the expansion of global health: the speeding up of the
circulation of capital, knowledge, and technology, aimed to eliminate spatial barriers to access medical treatment, could be sustained only through physical and
social infrastructures that froze productive forces into a fixed spatial formation.[17]
Inspired by the writings of philosopher Peter Sloterdijk on capital, technology,
and form, I will later describe this spatial formation as an archipelago of care and

expertise.[18] PAN did not emulate the kind of distributed, rhizomatic organization often associated with global capitalism—and indeed with global health—and its compulsions to connect and liberate flows.[19] Rather, it organized emerging connections alongside enduring patterns of circulation and exclusion. One of the primary challenges posed by PAN is to try to think about connectivity *with* insulation in contemporary global capitalism, including in the design of medical worlds. The challenge also is to think about both the indeterminacy of the futures created by PAN and the narrowing of the field of possibilities inherent to expectations associated with PAN as a project and a gift—more on this in chapter 4.

The Gift—From the South

"We're a nation of a billion people and our thought is: 'What can I give to the world?'" explained Dr. Abdul Kalam when we met at his 10 Rajaji Marg residence in New Delhi in March 2011. "We can give knowledge. We can remove the pain of the people. That is that type of culture we have," continued Kalam. The former president of India then recalled how it all began. It started with his presidential visit to South Africa, where he attended a session of the Pan-African Parliament in 2004. All of the African nations were represented, Kalam insisted. In his inaugural address, he engaged the audience with what he described as a vision: "Then the idea came in. How to connect them. Our hospitals and the African hospitals, our universities and the African universities, how we can connect? And when I presented, they cheered."

During the year before meeting with President Kalam, I'd had numerous discussions with Indian foreign affairs officers, project designers, and entrepreneurs involved in the early days, design, and implementation of PAN. In the course of these meetings, I had heard the story over and over again: PAN was a genuinely Indian contribution to the world and to Africa in particular. It was not, my interlocutors insisted, the type of project Western stakeholders would fund. My interlocutors seldom referred to the contemporary uptake of digital health in Western-centric global health spheres—for instance, to investments, policies, and reports by institutions such as the World Health Organization (WHO), the Bill and Melinda Gates Foundation, or the World Bank. Neither would they speak the language of aid or assistance—at times bluntly distancing themselves from approaches considered to be paternalistic. Western-centric agendas, institutions, and moral economies were not, here, key points of reference.

PAN drew attention to often neglected genealogies of trade and development, invoking the memory of earlier forms of South-South cooperation, including between India and Africa. Imaginations of the future, in PAN, mobilized narratives of technological humanism and political solidarity that have infused Indian claims of cooperation with Africa for many decades. PAN, as material infrastructure and political intervention, was not only looking toward the future: it was also built on top of the past. India-Africa relations have often become the object of a sanctimonious, quasi-mythical historiography that revolves around events such as the Bandung Conference or historical figures such as Jawaharlal Nehru and Mohandas Gandhi. For the designers of future India-Africa cooperation, a project like PAN subscribed to Gandhi's call for India and Africa to develop a form of commerce that would be "of ideas and services, not of manufactured goods against raw materials after the fashion of the Western exploiters" (Bhattacharya 2010, 63). But despite Gandhi's lasting moral ascendancy, the modern origins of an "Indian model" of cooperation with Africa are best found in Jawaharlal Nehru's engagement with the "sister continent." As will be examined in chapter 1, Nehru's engagement with Africa aimed to craft a uniquely Indian cooperation in which claims of difference and universality, past and future, were deeply entangled. On the one hand, for Nehru, India's capacity to come up with a distinct voice in world affairs was entrenched in its anciently rooted civilizational identity (Nehru 1961). Such an identity would give moral direction to the nation's contribution to the world and produce an Indian brand of South-South cooperation. On the other hand, for Nehru, South-South cooperation was a modern project, at once economic, political, and technoscientific.[20] South-South cooperation, in Nehruvian terms, would contest Western economic and technoscientific monopoly by cultivating a sense of solidarity. But it would do so by performing what Dipesh Chakrabarty (2005, 4812) referred to as "pedagogical politics" that enacts civilizational and cultural hierarchies, including between nations. India's approach to South-South cooperation was always concerned with performing the nation as a mentor and a global hub for knowledge and technology. The story of PAN is a modernist, capitalist, yet unmistakably Indian story.

In the months preceding President Kalam's vision of PAN, in 2004, the Hindu-nationalist-led state government instigated a radical shift in India's approach to international cooperation. As chapter 1 explains, the Indian state would soon drastically reduce the country's dependence on external donors and expand the lending of grants or project assistance to other developing countries. Over the course of the next few years, India would go from being the world's largest recipient of foreign aid to becoming a net donor. This came with significant investment by the Indian state aimed at fostering trade and cooperation with Africa. There was a refinancing of the long-standing Indian Technical and Economic Cooperation (ITEC) scheme, lines of credit programs were implemented to expand Indian exports to the African continent, and new diplomatic channels were established, culminating in the creation of the India–Africa Forum Summit.

It is therefore not a coincidence that PAN was launched in Africa instead of in neighboring South Asian countries, for example.[21] These years witnessed a rapid acceleration of bilateral trade between India and Africa, jumping from US$5.3 billion in 2001 to US$62 billion in 2018. India became Africa's third-largest trading partner behind China and the United States and the fourth-largest exporter of products to sub-Saharan Africa.[22] Health care and telecommunications, both of which were converging in PAN, are priority sectors for the expansion of Indian products and services. The rapid rise in the export of low-priced Indian pharmaceuticals to African countries and the Global South in general has been relatively well documented in recent years.[23] As was noted by Anne Pollock (2019, 128), India is often referred to as the "pharmacy of the developing world" by global health organizations. But the global expansion of India's medical industry in Africa also includes the outsourcing of medical services, rapidly growing medical tourism, and the spread of Indian private hospitals across the continent—all of which were actively pursued in PAN.

This book explores the conditions under which India and Africa are weaving the paths that tie both regions in the present and in the future (Mbembe 2012). "We *need* Africa but then what is the plan of action from the government?"[24] explained a high official at the Federation of Indian Chambers of Commerce and Industry (FICCI) when we met at the trade organization's headquarters. "There is a lack of interest. We are only a shadow of what China is doing." The reference to China is not trivial. In the many discussions I had with Indian entrepreneurs, state officials, and industry advocates, it became clear that a revitalized "Indian model" would have to take shape in contradistinction to "what China is doing" or is perceived as doing. As the narrative goes, the Chinese approach to the African continent is all about resource extraction, the export of cheap labor, and basic infrastructure projects such as buildings and roads. While PAN stakeholders have little to say about Western-centric interventions in Africa, they strongly insist that their approach is unlike China's. PAN instantiates such a claim. The aesthetics of networking, evoked in PAN's very title, comes with a sense of technological sophistication that can be understood as a rejection of the Chinese focus on "basic infrastructure projects." It also suggests an interest in alliances and connections, differentiating the network from a Chinese strategy perceived as self-serving, if not underhanded. Such othering of China by Indian stakeholders, along with rejections of Western-centric models of development, is often accompanied by claims of the South as a moral, economic, and political category. Over the past few years, significant attention has been given to how claims made about or in the name of the South—generally under the notions of the Global South or South-South cooperation—may challenge established economic orders and bring about new geopolitical affinities (Hofmeyr 2018; Menon 2018). Importantly, PAN did not position itself in relation to hegemonic centers: it conceived of the Global South as a market and medical formation of its own.

"It looks extremely well. It is good marketing,"[25] expressed a senior officer at the African Union Commission (AUC) when we met in Addis Ababa in 2011. "No one can refuse. You can't say 'no' to health, especially when it's free. So it's the best way to make an extraordinary breakthrough into the market," he continued. For some of my African interlocutors, PAN introduced an appealing alternative to the enduring influence of past colonial powers. It was certainly worth giving it a try. For PAN's participants, however, it was always obvious that the gift came with expectations of reciprocity. After all, the senior officer explained, the Indians competed with the Chinese in Africa. The analysis was straightforward but not condemnatory. PAN, suggested the AUC officer, was the product of a "brilliant reflection."

By mobilizing the South as a category, PAN promoted the expansion of Indian corporate hospitals as part of a win-win scenario: hospitals would reach a new patient base while patients got access to affordable treatment. Over the past decade, Indian hospitals have been actively branding themselves as capable of providing high-end health care at a fraction of the price of competing destinations or service providers. Health benefits are to be garnered alongside commercial profits, "displacing older critiques of profits' inevitable trade-offs for health" (Adams et al. 2019, 7). Health care and market potential are intertwined for good. In PAN, the South made the expansion of the Indian medical industry into a project of care and cooperation. Historical processes of differentiation and hierarchization—for instance, between Indian and African medical worlds—were branded as a market opportunity.

Cooperation in PAN did not carry the kind of promises of emancipation found in early forms of South-South solidarity. PAN, however, was not simply an expression of global capitalism. It was also the heir to complicated national and regional histories with their own scales and affective resonances. Contemporary and historical rivalry with China, for example, undermines the idea of a monolithic South. Most importantly, PAN disputed the still prevalent image of India as a recipient of global health interventions and expertise. In PAN, India emerged as the source and driving force behind another medical globalization, exporting biomedicine and hospital care. But what new market and medical formations do claims of South-South cooperation enable (McKay 2019)? I argue that as a gift from the South, PAN performed a moral defense of an Indian brand of capitalism, thus legitimizing the expansion of global capital (Aneja 2015). But, in doing so, the network also substantiated claims about the conditions under which India and Africa should be included in a future world order. It came with expectations about the conditions under which the nation should *arrive* on the global stage.[26]

In PAN, the lines between market and gift exchange were often blurred. PAN was a vehicle for speculation on future medical markets. It also was a flamboyant gift, bound to remake the identities of giver and receiver, caregiver and patient, master and student.[27] As such, it opened up future possibilities that at least partially emerged from the past.

Capitalist Dreams, Technoscientific Futures

Having worked for the Indian Space Research Organization (ISRO) for over twenty years, President Kalam did not have to look very far to imagine what a uniquely Indian contribution to the world should look like. When he announced PAN in 2004, Kalam was well aware of the emergence of telemedicine in India over the previous decade. Since around the turn of the millennium, ISRO had indeed been using satellite technology to lay out a nationwide network connecting patients, medical practitioners, hospitals, and mobile units in all corners of a vast national territory.[28] At the moment PAN was launched, hundreds of medical centers were already connected to its network. ISRO was also a strong advocate for furthering the adoption of telemedicine in India. But what was being extended in all corners of the country was not merely a physical network. It was a *model* for the large-scale provision of medical care.

Telemedicine in India was deployed in line with ISRO's societal mission, which has become a trademark of the space agency since its inception in 1969: "harnessing space technology for national development."[29] Satellite technology, according to such a conception of national development, was to be put in the service of the common man. In the words of Vikram Sarabhai, the first chairperson of the Indian National Committee for Space Research—which would become ISRO in 1969—in 1962, the primary impact of satellite technology should not be a spectacle of "grandiose schemes" but rather "progress measured in hard economic and social terms" (cited in Harvey 2000, 130). It was thus following such a Nehruvian philosophy that, starting in the 1970s, ISRO initiated various tele-education programs and remote sensing applications aimed at tackling the real-life problems of the common man.

It was not until around the turn of the millennium, however, that telemedicine rapidly expanded in India. As chapter 1 examines, telemedicine then came to be seen as *the* appropriate technology to provide health care expertise to rural and remote populations in India. The deployment of telemedicine in India concurred with disinvestment in public health infrastructures. Telemedicine indeed imposed itself in the context of a growing disparity in health care access between urban and rural areas, which was largely the outcome of the privatization of India's hospital landscape in the aftermath of the neoliberal reforms implemented in the 1990s.[30] Policy documents such as the Tenth Five Year Plan of the Planning Commission of India, approved in 2002, for example, presented telemedicine as an acceptable solution to increasingly fragmented and unevenly distributed health care access. Satellite technology in particular promised to integrate primary health centers (PHCs) and district hospitals into a network of private tertiary-care hospitals.

In the first decade of the millennium, ISRO played a central role in the development of a nationwide telemedicine network in India. ISRO's engagement in telemedicine marked a shift from its previous socially inclined state-building program toward an entrepreneurial experiment in development and market creation. Telemedicine in India primarily spread through a series of public-private partnerships (PPP) between the Indian state—here, ISRO—and corporate hospitals such as forerunner Apollo Hospitals, whose telemedicine program was launched in 1999. The model was straightforward: while ISRO expanded and maintained the satellite network infrastructure free of cost, corporate hospitals would provide free medical teleconsultations. For rapidly growing hospital chains, telemedicine was—and still is—a tool to build a presence in semiurban, rural, and remote areas, thus facilitating access to new patients and places. Telemedicine, explained Dr. Prathap C. Reddy, chairman of Apollo Hospitals, in 2001, would vertically integrate the medical facility of the country (Business Line 2001). In such a vertically integrated health infrastructure, corporate chains gained remote access to new patients, who would often end up traveling to their facilities for treatment, without having to open hospitals in rural and remote areas. Telemedicine, however, does not simply respond to preexisting patient populations. It produces new remote patient populations, disentangled from the state as a care provider. The spread of telemedicine in India operates as a style of health and resource management that assembles pools of clients in profitable catchment regions (Cartwright 2000). Telemedicine turns splintered health care infrastructure and distance from services into a market opportunity. What is at stake is a modeling of statecraft in corporate and entrepreneurial terms.[31] In telemedicine, the state materializes on the ground "as both a deliberate absence and an imagined presence" (Adams et al. 2019, 5).

For telemedicine advocates, digital media promise to overcome the complications inherent to a national health system widely considered to be failing. Any obstruction in the flow of data and information is seen as an obstacle to the effective provision of medical care—leading to long and costly travel, if not to lack of access to care, suffering, and loss of life. Conversely, poor access to health care but also insecurity and precariousness are recast as informational issues: as digital divides that only an increase in connectivity might help bridge, beyond state-centric forms of social obligation.[32] What emerged in India around the turn of the millennium is a politics of care in which the valuation of life—as amenable to medical care—is not correlated with colocalization but rather with being connected and reachable at a distance.

The expansion of telemedicine in India is harnessed to capitalist dreams of market creation but also to the national imagination of technoscientific futures. Telemedicine sites in India are the object of massive affective and imaginative investments. They are frequently visited by diplomats, entrepreneurs, reporters, and foreign politicians. Media events are often staged on their premises. ISRO's development of satellite technology is often referred to as a postcolonial success story, a technocentric model of development that other countries from the Global South might want to emulate. The deployment of satellite technology for telemedicine, however, also fires one's imagination for future economic growth. The promise of the satellite in the 2000s had to be situated within a broader economy of hope in which digital technology, capital, and the nation were closely intertwined. Indeed, in the years preceding PAN's launch, digital connectivity was being celebrated as a source of empowerment, greater productivity, improved governance, and nation-building in India. As the narrative went, after decades of suffering from a series of structural bureaucratic and political obstructions, digital media were to release long-suppressed entrepreneurial and technoscientific energies.[33] Weaving together reminiscences of past glory and dreams of coming prosperity, they seemed to unlock a sense of possibility and rising aspirations.[34] They would also become central to the recognition of the nation's growth story by global capital and to the "nation branding" project for twenty-first-century India.[35] *Life at a Distance* examines the materializing force of this project.

The Mother of All Networks

> But what I do know is that there is no greater power in heaven or on earth than the commitment to a dream. Dreams hold something of that energy which lies at the heart of all things and are the binding force that brings the spiritual and the material together.
>
> —APJ Abdul Kalam (2003, 19)

The notion that telemedicine can reconfigure access to medical care is not unique to India. Over the past decade, digital technology has attracted much attention from the global health community as a technological solution that can short-circuit inadequate health infrastructure. Be it in war zones, in humanitarian contexts, or as part of development policies, interventions relying on digital technology to provide medical care and monitoring are proliferating in low- and middle-income countries. Academic literature, institutional publications, industry reports, and advocacy papers have also been praising the "transformative power" of electronic media, suggesting critical changes in the management of patient care on a global scale.[36] The appeal of digital technology in global health, however, has been partially offset in recent years by rampant criticism of limited evidence of its durable impact on health outcomes.[37] Noting that a majority of projects are failing to move beyond the pilot stage, the question is now raised with urgency by stakeholders: How can networks grow durably? How can they scale or integrate existing medical systems? While responses to these important questions differ, there is a growing consensus within global health spheres according to which, if it is to fulfill its promises, digital health must produce robust data about what works and what does not, as well as about which interventions are deemed valuable and should be scaled.[38] In congruence with narratives and practices that are dominant in global health, the expansion of digital health apparently should depend upon reliable data, metrics, and standards.[39] Put simply, it should be based on scientific knowledge and evidence.

"You have to think big. Dr. Kalam, he thinks big. It was his vision!"[40] explained a former TCIL executive when we met in New Delhi in 2011. PAN, the manager asserted, was not a one-off initiative. It was a catalyst: seeing the success of this project, many more projects would come to life. The network, he suggested, would inevitably multiply: "It's the mother of all telemedicine projects." PAN was to act as an incubator for future relations. Its designers and sponsors were thus also preoccupied with questions of growth. But their position vis-à-vis the proper conditions for a digital health network to expand and produce new relations contrasted sharply with global health demands for accounting, metrics, and evidence. Numbers never played a key role in the way the project justified its existence. For PAN's stakeholders, metrics were not the appropriate way to assess its impact. Building relations, for PAN, was never a question of good measure. It was, by contrast, a matter of excessive promises and deferral. Value in PAN was driven by speculation, not experimentation.

There are many ways to approach PAN's speculative logic. One would be to insist on the gap between the promise generated by PAN and its day-to-day workings and achievements. PAN provided medical care in uneven if not erratic ways. The quality of the services offered was inconsistent, largely because of discrepancies across sites in terms of the conditions under which care was made accessible and practiced. As chapter 5 examines, PAN was also heavily underutilized, especially when considering the sumptuary expenditure that it occasioned. A key reason for this lies in the design of the network, which did not attend or respond to stated needs. Put simply, local concerns and realities were largely ignored in the design of the network. As a scaling project, PAN carried a strong universalizing impetus. By design, connected sites were rendered remote. PAN followed its own path, irrespective of the real needs of its participants. The kinds of dreams materially inscribed in the design of PAN thus ultimately stood as obstacles to the project's implementation and everyday life.

But merely underlining how PAN failed to be rolled out as planned and meet preset objectives would thus be missing the point: PAN was speculative in the sense that it *could not* have determined or known effects. Many of PAN's stakeholders displayed unwavering trust in the power of the network. For them, the network's capacity to build future relations was never compromised—it was only ever deferred. Deferral explained away any obstacle faced by the network, thus framing the obstacle as momentary, soon to be overcome. There was a sense that the project might not be rolled out as planned but would nevertheless eventually work its magic. PAN did not only speed up circulation between connected sites. It also introduced a *delay*.[41] The map may not have been the territory, as the saying goes. But it promised the territory. It just was not *yet* the territory.

PAN generated futures by putting together what Anna Tsing (2005) referred to as a conjuring or dramatic performance. Value, in PAN, was indissociable from attracting attention. The network, for instance, came with a world of business representatives, ritualized diplomatic touring, and photo opportunities. From its very beginnings, it benefited from extensive public exposure. It received substantial media coverage both in India and in Africa. Politicians and high-ranking government officials would often visit the network's premises. PAN was awarded prestigious prizes. Corporate films were released about PAN, gleaming with images of modern technology, fake patients, and promises of economic miracles. Appearances were also carefully crafted in countless brochures, flyers, political speeches, and official declarations or statements.

A key feature of PAN's dramatization of the world was to be found in the charismatic energy of Dr. Abdul Kalam himself. Dr. Kalam, who passed away in 2015, was a larger-than-life scientist, icon, and leader in India, well beyond telemedicine spheres. Kalam was widely referred to as the "People's President" or the "Missile Man of India," nicknames respectively denoting his humble origins and his role in India's nuclear program. Kalam displayed the magical ability to connect with people and inspire India's youth in ways that cut across ethnic, religious, caste, and class lines. As STS scholar Shiv Visvanathan (2015) noted, Kalam was a "performative spectacle" in which people wanted to believe. Researching PAN, I rapidly came to realize that attachment to PAN was inseparable from attachment to Kalam. Just like the satellite, Kalam imparted the nation with a sense of future possibility.[42] Once again, however, it was the *past* that served as the primary indicator of what the future held. Kalam's vision was one in which the nation rediscovered itself as a strong and sovereign land of knowledge (Kalam 2003, 121). PAN would therefore contribute to restoring an ancient order of things with India occupying, at last, her "rightful place on this planet" (Kalam 2011, 107). In doing so, it also reimagined the place of Africa and India within global capitalism. Building new relations, for PAN, was thus never an issue of methodical expansion based on metrics or evidence but rather a matter of speculation: of imagining worlds into existence. How, after all, would one ever quantify the persuasive power of a vision?

Traces

Over the past decade, I have been tracking the Pan-African e-Network, mostly in India but also in Dakar (Senegal) and Addis Ababa (Ethiopia). In 2010–11, a few years after PAN was launched, I spent large amounts of time in the participating hospitals. The network was connecting twelve hospitals, all of which were located in urban areas. Corporate hospitals such as Fortis Hospital (Noida) and Narayana Hrudayalaya (Bangalore) were connected alongside iconic institutions such as the All India Institute of Medical Sciences (New Delhi) or Dr. Balabhai Nanavati Hospital (Mumbai). I have spent time and conducted interviews in eight of the twelve participating Indian hospitals. This provided me with a sense of the network's scale as well as of the infrastructure and labor sustaining its everyday operations. Most importantly, I have benefited from prolonged stays in two hospitals that occupied a prominent position in PAN—namely, Apollo Hospital in Chennai and CHNU Fann in Dakar.

Located in the heart of the southern Indian metropolis, also the capital of Tamil Nadu, the Apollo Hospital in Chennai was founded in 1983. It was the first hospital of the Apollo group, which would later become a key player in the privatization of the Indian hospital sector starting in the 1990s. By the time PAN was launched in 2009, Apollo's hospital in Chennai boasted over 1,000 beds spread over 60 departments. Apollo Hospitals was the largest hospital chain in India, with over 8,500 beds across 50 hospitals in India. It had also recently opened its first hospital in Mauritius, with the ambition to open many more hospitals in Africa. Under the leadership of Dr. Krishnan Ganapathy, Apollo had also been playing a key role in the growth of telemedicine in India since the turn of the millennium. It was hardly surprising, then, that Apollo's hospital in Chennai would soon become an active participant in PAN: over the first two years of PAN activities, the hospital had been involved in 170 teleconsultations on the network—a considerable amount given PAN's generally poor utilization. *Life at a Distance* draws on the months I spent at Apollo Hospital in Chennai. The same holds true for the CHNU Fann in Dakar. When deciding how I should track PAN's activities in Africa, CHNU Fann soon appeared as the best place to start. Fann was one of the primary users of the network. While I was attending medical teleconsultations from India, I would sometimes have discussions with Fann's engineers and doctors.[43] This was facilitated by the fact that French is my native language. During the months spent at Fann, I also realized that the hospital was serious about telemedicine. Under the leadership of Dr. Bara Diop, a team of engineers was working to implement telemedicine services across the country in addition to participating in PAN. This provided me an opportunity to spend time with people who were capable of and earnest about making PAN work and to observe some of its concrete effects.

A significant portion of this research has involved retracing the history and materiality of PAN, both as an idea and as a thing. My interest in the aesthetics and promises held by PAN has also led me to attend a large variety of events where it was being staged. This includes conferences, trade exhibitions, and political spectacles. In events like the India–Africa Forum Summit (IAFS), Telemedicon (the annual international conference of the Telemedicine Society of India), and the Ethio Health Exhibition and Congress in Addis Ababa, one could get a good sense of the desires that were being invested in the network. These events were also occasions to meet with senior government officials, entrepreneurs, managers, industry advocates, and politicians—all of whom believed, for all sorts of reasons, in the power of the network. But *Life at a Distance* also exposes the much less visible infrastructural layers, protocols, and material fabrics that supported the network *from below*. It makes visible the labor, materiality, and operations that remained concealed or unnoticed, contrasting with the public attention that the project captured (Harvey, Jensen, and Morita 2016). This was primarily done by spending time in PAN's studios and data centers, including TCIL's data center and headquarters in New Delhi and the Hub Center on the outskirts of Dakar. PAN engineers, working from within connected hospitals, became key interlocutors, if not friends. I was also fortunate enough to count key actors involved in the design and implementation of PAN as interlocutors. Meetings with space scientists from ISRO provided me with a better sense of the technology and the vision inscribed into the design of the network. I also had access to a vast number of documents detailing the history, design, and implementation of the network. Annual reports, technical blueprints, films, flyers, five-year plans, industry forecasts, and private PowerPoint presentations were instrumental in tracing the shape of the network.

Structure of the Book

Life at a Distance is composed of five chapters, an introduction, and a short epilogue. Chapter 1 recounts PAN's manifold histories, seeking to understand how it came to be considered "a shining example of South-South cooperation," or, in the words of President Kalam, as India's "gift to the world." The chapter recounts past iterations of cooperation between Africa and India, whether it be in events such as the Bandung Conference, programs such as the Indian Technical and Economic Cooperation (ITEC), or moral philosophies such as *vasudhaiva kutumbakam*. PAN did not carry the kind of redemptive hopes found in early forms of Afro-Asian solidarity. PAN embodied a key shift in India's approach to South-South cooperation, moving away from Nehruvian socialist humanism toward a conception of cooperation as an economic opportunity. Chapter 1 shows how a key challenge, in tracing PAN's genealogies, is to differentiate between enduring *ideas* of South-South solidarity and the historical processes effectively shaping postcolonial relations between India and Africa (Vitalis 2013). The aim is not so much to distinguish real versus imagined relations. Rather, it is to try to explore the effects of claiming the South as a speculative project.

Addressing these questions also entails recounting the fascinating story of telemedicine in India. Chapter 1 shows how telemedicine in India was born out of the social, modernist mission of ISRO. ISRO's pioneering use of satellite technology for development purposes can be traced back as early as the 1970s. However, the chapter suggests that India's nationwide telemedicine network, supported by ISRO, also concurred with massive disinvestment in public health infrastructures. Telemedicine in India was primarily driven by the rise of corporate hospitals in the wake of the neoliberal reforms that transformed the health care landscape in India in the 1990s. Put roughly, telemedicine expanded as an experimental *model* for market creation and the provision of medical care at a distance. Chapter 1 examines the history of this model, which PAN incorporated and, indeed, exported.

Drawing upon ethnographic work, chapter 2 documents the materials, labor, and technical processes that composed PAN's network infrastructure. Through the presentation of patient cases, it also examines practices of mediation between remote clinical worlds. Chapter 2 describes PAN's sites, its actors, its equipment, and how it operated on an everyday basis. It examines how PAN's design is reflecting the recent history, at once infrastructural, economic, and political, of global connectivity. Particular attention is given to the history of PAN's material infrastructure, which combined optical fiber submarine communications cable systems and satellite technology. In dialogue with STS and media studies work, the chapter also shows how care practices were embedded in and supported by labor practice. It documents the work of the engineers who were dispatched all over India and Africa to take care of the network and sustain its operations. Special attention is given to the network's everyday routine, which was often at odds with the temporalities of accelerated flows and circulation generally associated with digital technology. Attention to infrastructure and labor practices presents a case against the temptation to fetishize—if not naturalize—global flows of capital, knowledge, and technology.

Chapter 3 examines how PAN produced networked medical enclosures. It attends to the network's topology and the control exerted over the circulation of knowledge over the network. PAN, I suggest, enacted tensions between emergent global flows and unchanging spatial forms. PAN was enclaved by design: it was organizationally, spatially, and technically isolated from the hospitals it connected. The network's studios were located in secluded spaces reserved for the sole purpose of telemedicine. They were not integrated within care units and were isolated from their daily activities. Enclaves were also clinical. Chapter 3 describes patient cases that illustrate how digital health can lead to or reinforce patterns of enclosure that shape access to medical care on a global scale. In dialogue with scholarship on medicine, space, and technology—starting with Michel Foucault's writings on the clinic—the chapter examines how telemedicine makes certain people and things more visible than others. PAN made remote peoples and sites into objects of medical intervention. But chapter 3 shows how, in doing so, it also structured the circulation of medical knowledge in specific ways, reified distinctions among peoples and places, and enacted tensions between opening and closure, territorialization, and deterritorialization (Mbembe 2018).

Chapter 4 examines the speculative logic that animated PAN as a commercial, moral, and political project. PAN was indeed the object of great affective and financial investment. PAN produced value by staging dramatic performances of imagined futures and collectivities. As is often the case with telemedicine, many considered PAN an investment in accelerated market exchange. The network was to help Indian health care providers build a commercial presence on the African continent. It would accelerate the flow of knowledge but also patients, technology, and capital between India and Africa. PAN was not designed for short-term profit. It did not in itself generate a sustainable stream of revenue. Rather, the network created value by building trust in *future* medical and commercial relations between participants. Hospital managers, for sure, hoped to see their brand name circulate and their patient base expand. However, a key argument developed in this chapter is that attachments to PAN went beyond economic rationality. The network acted as a medium for the nation to perform itself as an emergent global health and technological power. Through PAN, remote interventions into the lives of other peoples shaped the imagination of the nation. Ultimately, chapter 4 explores aesthetic, material, and political forms shaping contemporary India as the empire of speculation.[44]

Chapter 5 examines some of the challenges encountered by PAN. Obstacles to PAN's flourishing were indeed plenty. At times, equipment was being held up at customs or redistributed within hospitals for other purposes. There were also communication barriers, whether linguistic or technical. In many hospitals, there was a lack of awareness of the project. TCIL officers blamed African doctors for not using the network enough or encouraging their colleagues to do so. By contrast, doctors in African hospitals insisted that PAN did not take into consideration their needs, schedules, or working conditions. As a result, using the network was often seen as a challenging if not aggravating experience. Chapter 5 suggests that PAN's speculative logic undermined the conditions for its existence in the present. The desire for rapid, seamless expansion compromised the messy mediation work required for a project like PAN to be viable.

In writing this book, I had no interest in providing a full representation of PAN. The book does not aim to stitch together bits and pieces that might illuminate otherwise invisible materials, spaces, and processes to provide a coherent picture. Rather, my aim was to cultivate an ethnographic practice that breaks open totalizing abstractions and interrogates the assumed coherence, durability, or knowability of shared social worlds (Biehl and Locke 2017; Wool and Livingston 2017). *Life at a Distance* makes visible the glitches, failures to communicate, passing time, political passions, and absent users—all of which are not external to but rather constitutive of the network.[45] Ethnographic inquiry complicates fantasies of a unified sphere of communication, expressed in images such as the satellite footprint. It challenges a connectionist conception of networking in which what is communicated could be severed from *how* it is communicated. To dreams of closure and finitude, *Life at a Distance* prefers the opacities that coexist and weave the network's fabrics. But this in turn raises a thorny question: How can ethnography maintain itself in the right relationship with such opacities?[46] In researching PAN and preparing this manuscript, I have found that a key challenge was to avoid the kind of closures that would emulate PAN's homogenizing motive, driven by a coherent promise or vision. To a large extent, this was done by sitting in the middle of the gap between the promises and realities of PAN. A related challenge, however, was to do so without falling for a facile, dismissive cynicism about the dreams and passions invested in PAN. I never believed it was mine to decide whether PAN was a success or a failure, a good or a bad project. Rather, I was interested in how PAN intervened in the world and to what effect. My aim has been to excavate the materialities, practices, and forms of power that shaped the inner spaces of the network in all their turbulence, splendor, and inadequacies. This book can also be read as a kind of speculation of its own on the commercial, political, and moral value being conjured in PAN. Of what futures, I have kept wondering, could such a project be the harbinger?

A SHINING EXAMPLE

A shining example of South-South cooperation.
—Slogan of the Pan-African e-Network

Space technology in the service of humankind.
—Motto of the Indian Space Research Organisation (ISRO)

Two months after President Kalam had the vision of PAN, on November 5, 2004, Manmohan Singh inaugurated the Hindustan Times Leadership Initiative Conference in New Delhi with the theme India and the World: A Blueprint for Partnership and Growth. The newly elected prime minister of India was speaking in front of a distinguished audience, which included the former US secretary of state Henry Kissinger as a guest of honor. The world, suggested Singh in an explicit reference to the conference's prosaic title, expected an "ancient, civilizational nation" like India to "bring to the table of global discourse something more than strategic partnerships and market opportunities" (Singh 2004). India's unique contribution to the world, Singh explained, was rather to be found in her intellectual history and in her moral and political disposition to offer an alternative to binary thinking (us/them) and especially to the idea of a "clash of civilizations" that would go against the "true spirit of our ancient land" (Singh 2004).

Prime Minister Singh's address can be understood as a direct rebuttal to Henry Kissinger's vision, in which the establishment of world order leaves little place for moral considerations and in which, as Kissinger infamously suggested, "Nothing important can come from the South."[1] Singh insisted that a genuinely Indian understanding of the world shall envision it as a "global family," an idea that he traced back to an age-old philosophical tradition: "The idea of unity in diversity, drawing on the wisdom of our forefathers who spoke of vasudhaiva kutumbakam—that translates as 'The Whole World Is One Family'" (Singh 2004). The notorious Sanskrit saying vasudhaiva kutumbakam, Singh reminded the audience, had inspired the Indian freedom struggle, and it best illustrated the many-sidedness and cooperative pluralism upon which India's approach to world affairs was built: "unity in diversity." According to Singh, vasudhaiva kutumbakam was a powerful yet practical political basis for dealing with the most daunting challenges of our times and could thus be considered India's most precious gift to the world.[2]

Giving historical and historiographical credence to his metaphysical musings, Prime Minister Singh soon moved on to quote Jawaharlal Nehru, who, in The Discovery of India, famously called for the nation to "come out of her shell and take full part in the life and activities of the modern age" (Nehru 2004, 619). The reference to Nehru is hardly surprising. Prime minister and foreign minister of India from Independence in 1947 to his death in 1964, Nehru was the main architect of the country's foreign policy. Similar to Manmohan Singh, Nehru liked to insist on how India's unique civilizational identity should be instrumental in crafting a distinct voice in world affairs.[3] However, as we shall later see, the importance of such ancient-rooted civilizational wisdom in Nehru's brand of internationalism paled in comparison to claims for cooperation that were resolutely liberal and cosmopolitan (Sharma 2012). The reference to Nehru—and indeed Singh's whole speech—nevertheless drew attention to the complex entanglement, shaping India's imagination of her role in world affairs, between claims of difference and universality, specifically between metaphysically ridden notions of civilizational identity and the practical imagination of open-ended futures whose ultimate form remains to be determined.[4]

Interestingly, Manmohan Singh delivered his philosophical musings about India's place in world affairs only a few weeks after India's President Abdul Kalam had announced the creation of the Pan-African e-Network during a visit to South Africa. As mentioned in the introduction, Kalam had imagined PAN as a response to a question very similar to the one raised by Singh: What could India's gift to the world be? But how did a transnational network infrastructure aimed at providing medical care at a distance come to be seen as the appropriate gift to the world? This chapter examines this question by retracing the historical, material, and affective conditions of possibility of the Pan-African e-Network.

~~~

"The first principle of India's involvement in Africa is unlike that of China. China says 'go out and exploit the natural resources,' our strategy is to add value," suggested the Indian minister of state for commerce Jairam Ramesh during the India–Africa Forum Summit held in New Delhi in 2008 (cited in Vines 2010, 5). At first sight, Ramesh's comparison might appear particularly bold. But it summarizes a widespread narrative in Indian business spheres, according to which India's brand of South-South cooperation shall distinguish itself not primarily from a Western one but more importantly from China's. Put simply, corporate India considers itself in competition with China in Africa at both economic and moral levels. The many consultants, entrepreneurs, and officials in the Indian business spheres I spoke with during the course of my research for this book were adamant that Africa was the next frontier of economic growth for India. However, they also unanimously complained that in order for Indian companies to expand and crack new markets in Africa, there was a dire need for more support from the Indian state.

The Pan-African e-Network came as a response to these growing demands by Indian industries for better state support to facilitate access to new markets in Africa—thus allowing Indian industries to compete with China. "When China builds highways in exchange for oil supply, India does not have the means to follow and prefers to fall back on its Pan-African e-Network," suggested Patrick de Jac-quelot, a French correspondent in India, two years after the project was launched (de Jacquelot 2011, my translation). My Indian interlocutors were indeed keen to point out that PAN was precisely the type of network that *neither* Western donors nor the Chinese government would engage in. The former could provide aid or relief but could not deliver affordable and appropriate health services to African patients in a sustainable way. The latter is apparently all about brick and mortar, with overbearing governmental control. Because of its overreliance on govern-mental support, the Chinese strategy is perceived as self-serving, constraining Africa's future. A senior officer at the Confederation of Indian Industry explained to me, "The difference between the Chinese model and the Indian model is that the Indian model is more sustainable, developing local capacities. India has been a colony. So we understand those sensitive things better than some other countries. We want inclusive growth, not exploitative growth."[5]

The distinctiveness of India's approach is framed in civilizational, moral, and historical terms. When the time comes to emphasize the originality of the Indian model, past solidarities, imagined and real, are revived in contemporary South-South cooperation narratives.[6] They contain the seeds of cooperation to come. Pasts, presents, and futures, however, are not following each other in sequence: they coexist, as the past is taken to indicate what the future holds (Philip 2016, 279).

As this chapter will make clear, early South-South cooperation was associated with the possibility to challenge colonial power and its continuance as well as with dreams of a new world order. PAN, however, did not carry this kind of hope. Nor could it be associated with more recent calls to decolonize global health. It did not challenge and in fact may have amplified the kind of neoliberal econom-ics that has been guiding the development of global health over the past decades. After all, PAN was a state-sponsored project aimed at opening new markets for Indian private hospitals on the African continent. It accelerated the expansion of global capital and of the Indian medical industry in particular. As such, it could be seen as an illustration of what Vijay Prashad (2013, 10) refers to as the "South from above": neoliberalism with Southern characteristics. But reducing

PAN to a mimicry of the neoliberal global North is hardly satisfying. When taking seriously the civilizations narrative expressed by Manmohan Singh or Abdul Kalam—respectively, prime minister and president of India when the project was launched—it becomes obvious that PAN's capacity to make us imagine futures cannot be reduced to economic interests alone. Although the network was animated by commercial motivations, economic instrumentality indeed remained in the background to a large extent. It yielded to more grandiose nationalist-capitalist promises in India.[7] In PAN, the nation-brand carried some kind of sublime quality: something that can't be bought or sold. But as this chapter suggests, in sharp contrast with early promises of South-South cooperation, the nationalism expressed in PAN is no longer anticolonial but is rather an offensive, expansion-driven brand of technonationalism. This chapter shows how past and future dreams of the nation cohere within this expansion and materialize in PAN.

The Pan-African e-Network, then, was a gift. But it was not only giving care, knowledge, or technology. Traveling alongside the network was a *model* for social development—specifically, for the distribution of health care and knowledge—at a distance. This model was developed in India in the form of a nationwide experiment in telemedicine. This chapter retraces the emergence of telemedicine in India in the years preceding PAN, when space technology was harnessed in an attempt to reduce health care inequity in rural areas and new patient populations—and markets—for corporate hospitals located in urban areas were created. It suggests that PAN, as a gift, aimed to remodel not only the distribution of biomedicine on a global scale but also, in doing so, the very identity of donor and recipient—making Africa the place where the Indian model, and indeed the nation itself, gets projected. PAN stood for anticipated, unrealized futures: fertile grounds from which hopes, dreams, and desires were to arise.[8]

Bandung Dreams—And Beyond

On April 18, 1955, Jawarharlal Nehru arrived in the town of Bandung, Indonesia, to attend the first large-scale Asian-African Conference. Over the next couple of days, delegates from twenty-nine countries in Asia and Africa, most of which were newly independent states, convened in what is now popularly known as the Bandung Conference. The explicit aim of the conference was to promote Afro-Asian economic and cultural cooperation and to oppose colonialism and neocolonialism. Prominent world leaders including Nehru, Indonesian president Sukarno, Egyptian president Nasser, and Chinese premier Zhou Enlai gathered to discuss common challenges their nations faced in navigating a postcolonial world. The Bandung Conference is commonly recognized as a central moment in the period of decolonization after the Second World War. Bandung came with great significance for the decentering of the West and decoloniality.[9] As was noted by Quỳnh N. Phạm and Robbie Shilliam, the meeting was "remarkable insofar as it provided the first diplomatic space in twentieth-century international relations that promised an intimacy among colonized and postcolonized peoples" (2016, 6). Participants at Bandung announced that they were global actors in their own right, no longer to be "treated as the anonymous, obedient, or chaotic 'rest' in the shadow of the West" (13).

India was a legitimate aspirant to leadership in regional gatherings such as the Bandung Conference.[10] Bandung was an ideal stage for leaders such as Nehru to frame "Indianness" in relation to contemporary events and to ensure that India would take her pride of place in the global order of nations. At Bandung, the "voice" of Bharat-mata (Mother India) had an international audience (Chakrabarty 2005, 4815). As usual, Nehru displayed a studied mix of principles rooted in an ancient Indian way of life and a spirit of cooperation driven by a strong international ethos. Nehru liked to emphasize that India's foreign policy was to be rooted in civilizational distinctiveness, including philosophical and political traditions. For instance, he tried to root the Five Principles of Peaceful Coexistence, or Panscheel, which he promoted at the conference, in some ancient and Indian "way of life" (Vitalis 2013, 272). Insisting on India's unique civilization had the obvious advantage of challenging one of the central legitimations of colonial rule—namely, the "superiority" of Western civilization.[11] It opened up new perspectives on the past, the present, and the future. However, the nationalism practiced by Nehru remained outward-looking and anticolonial.[12] For example, engagement with Africa was a top priority for Nehru to the extent that African decolonization was the continuation of India's own anticolonial struggles. Nehru's ideological reclaiming of vasudhaiva kutumbakam as part of a story of civilizational difference, therefore, has to be situated in the context of the fight against colonial expansion: the unity expressed by vasudhaiva kutumbakam was weaponized as a *response* to the imperialism of the West.[13] Nehru's well-known commitment to human rights and the "freedom of the common man" was thus entirely contingent upon economic and political liberation.

Just like Nehru, no one had any doubt at Bandung about the fact that the continued existence of colonialism and racial discrimination was the principal problem of human rights in the world (Chatterjee 2016, 329). There was a shared sense that the capacity for recently colonized nations to claim their space in world affairs entailed the refusal of cultural suppression and economic subordination (Prashad 2013, 45–46). Hence Bandung's final communiqué opened with the desire for greater economic cooperation in the Asian-African region.[14] The communiqué then moved on to underline the importance for participating countries to provide technical assistance to one another, including in the form of education and technical projects, and the exchange of know-how at regional scales. Such economic and technical cooperation would soon become the key feature around which India's approach to South-South cooperation would revolve. For Nehru, it was cooperation and collective self-reliance among the developing countries that would contribute to the establishment of a new economic order.

In addition to the realpolitik of such a new order in the making, Bandung also came with a strong affective dimension. Attachments to the so-called Bandung Spirit revealed an investment in anticolonial and decolonial affects, stimulating many peoples to challenge "the enduring archives of empire" (Agathangelou 2016, 103). In recent years, however, Bandung has at times become mythologized—in both scholarly work and popular or political renderings—as an example of a lost spirit of cooperation among newly independent Third World countries.[15] Nostalgic renditions of the event tend to present Bandung as a moment of unification around questions of race or color, or as the birthplace of the Non-Aligned Movement. Recent work has shown, however, that beyond the rhetoric of unity, Bandung was also a platform through which political tensions and opportunism emerged.[16] It reflected uneven processes of decolonization, geopolitical asymmetries, and competing national state-building projects.

India is a good example of this. When Nehru insisted, at Bandung, on Asia's duty "to help Africa to the best of her ability,"[17] he was also reaffirming that one continent was in a position to help and guide the other. At Bandung and elsewhere, Nehru aimed to inscribe his idea of Indianness onto India's regional spaces, including India-Africa, which defined the role that the Indian state was to play in such spaces (S. Singh 2011). As was suggested by Dipesh Chakrabarty, Nehru used the Bandung stage to perform a "pedagogical style of politics" in which the "very performance of politics re-enacted civilizational or cultural hierarchies: between nations, between classes, or between the leaders and the masses" (Chakrabarty 2005, 4812). Nehru's leadership at Bandung came with normative power: the norms and rules of international relations should be set in line with India's values (Hall 2017).

As a non-Western performance of self-determination, Bandung was nevertheless promoting a global system predicated on the nation-state. Each state would be responsible for the management of its own development. For instance, behind the pedagogical politics performed by Nehru was the "emergent and territorial nation state putting development ahead of diversity" (Chakrabarty 2005, 4815). In contrast with dreams of wholeness and unity, Nehru's conception of world affairs thus came with a sense—at times quite strong, at times much less so—of divergence, if not exceptionalism. As important as it might have been, unity was not the end goal in itself.[18]

Under such circumstances, South-South cooperation, including between India and Africa, was imagined as inextricably tied to a strong nation-building project. Nehru's vision of cooperation was nationalist and developmentalist in ways that contradict the somewhat romantic view of Bandung and indeed of South-South cooperation as a vehicle for horizontal solidarity.[19]

Central to the Nehruvian promise of cooperation was a formidable commitment to science, technology, and economic self-determination.[20] For Nehru, the modern state could literally be "produced" through scientific knowledge and technology (Abraham 1996, 325). Science and technology stood for authority and a higher form of knowledge. This also entailed a teleological view of social progress, according to which science and technology could in themselves determine whether a country was backward or developed. In other words, even though technoscientific cooperation did not, for Nehru, feed a parochial brand of nationalism, it favorably positioned the country along the hierarchy of national development. For a certain postcolonial Indian elite, then, technoscientific cooperation with Africa would both shape the imagination of the continent *and* revive the dream of India occupying its rightful place in the world. This dream is no doubt a key legacy of Nehru's version of South-South cooperation, which persists to this day. It is this very dream that would, decades later, materialize in the Pan-African e-Network.

Early Cooperation and Nation-Building

The Philosophy of ITEC flows from an age old ethos of Vasudhaiva Kutumbakam, which means the world is one big family.

—Advertising for the Indian Technical and Economic Cooperation Program

In the years following the conference, the "Bandung Spirit" translated into rather hesitant commitments to actual cooperation between India and Africa.[21] Throughout the 1950s, Nehru's government made modest attempts to provide technical support and training to countries such as Ethiopia and Egypt as well as the newly independent states of Ghana and Sudan. In addition, Nehru took it upon himself to ensure that places were reserved in Indian medical and engineering colleges for students from East Africa, at times personally intervening to ensure that tuition fees were maintained at an affordable level (Chhabra 1989). Consistent with the kind of collective self-reliance and socialist development he supported, Nehru was keen to put Indian economic, material, and political resources at the service of African independence (Prashad 2002, 143). The government of India's early South-South cooperation efforts also included participation in multilateral programs such as the Colombo Plan and the technical assistance program of the United Nations.[22] South-South cooperation on a large scale, however, would not be implemented until the mid-1960s, a few months after Nehru served his last days as prime minister of India.

On September 15, 1964, the cabinet of India made the decision to establish the Indian Technical and Economic Cooperation (ITEC) scheme. A bilateral assistance program, ITEC would remain the flagship of India's technoeconomic cooperation effort for the next four decades. With the launch of ITEC a few months after the passing of Nehru, India's economic cooperation went into high gear. The need to forge economic linkages among developing countries was first clearly articulated in the 1964–65 Annual Report of the External Affairs Ministry, where it was presented as an effort to fend off economic dependence on developed countries.[23] The aim of ITEC was to increase self-reliance in nation-building by meeting the demands of newly emerging states for technical support and trained personnel. However, the driving force of India's economic cooperation with Africa in the mid-1960s was primarily political. ITEC was born out of a political need to strengthen India's international presence and, more specifically, to counter China's ever-increasing aid diplomacy in Africa (Arbab 2006; Kragelund 2010; Singh 2010). The program was launched in the aftermath of the humiliating Sino-Indian War, when the downfall of India's influence and credibility on the African continent became glaringly obvious (Dubey 1991). Simultaneously, China was starting to gain influence given the substantial economic support it provided to African countries that sought financial and material assistance. It went beyond India's primarily diplomatic, moral, and rhetorical approach to cooperation.[24] For India, technoscientific cooperation was seen as an occasion to strengthen political ties in the context of nonalignment.

Throughout the 1970s and 1980s, India diversified its channels of cooperation with the African continent. Under Indira Gandhi's leadership, India provided financial and material assistance through mechanisms such as the OAU, the UN Fund for Namibia, the UN Educational and Training Programme for South Africa, and the Action for Resisting Invasion, Colonialism and Apartheid (AFRICA) fund. India's commitment to South-South cooperation was also channeled through the South Commission. Established in 1987 to continue the work of the worn-out Non-Aligned Movement, the South Commission was an intergovernmental grouping of developing countries in the South aiming to act as a countervailing power to the economic and intellectual hegemony of the North (Jain 2016). In the words of Manmohan Singh, then secretary-general of the South Commission, "The new locomotive forces have to be found within the South itself. South-South cooperation is, therefore, crucial" (Johny 2013).

In spite of these political attempts, for over four decades ITEC has remained— along with its corollary Special Commonwealth African Assistance Programme

(SCAAP)—the most practical component of India's South-South cooperation efforts, both in Africa and elsewhere. Since 1964, it has granted nearly $US2.5 billion in training and technical assistance to developing countries—out of which an estimated $US1 billion has gone to African states. Managed by the Ministry of External Affairs, ITEC allocates assistance using a system in which slots are exchanged for five different aid modalities: civilian training and defense training programs within Indian institutions; project-based cooperation; technical assistance (through the deputation of experts); study tours; and aid for disaster relief. While civilian training is the most important dimension, project-based cooperation extends to a variety of sectors and activities.[25] Sixty years after it was launched, ITEC is still operating in 160 countries, and its activities show no sign of abating.

In a scheme like ITEC, development was always meant to be put in the service of nation-building. Following a Nehruvian approach, India's early engagement in South-South cooperation revolved around a strong version of the nation-state.[26] Because he believed in the soundness of economic planning, Nehru maintained that socioeconomic emancipation was intrinsically dependent on the strengthening of national independence and political sovereignty. Having experienced the frustrations of economic dependency and subjugation under colonial rule, he thought of cooperation as a channel for enhanced self-reliance. The transnational circulation of knowledge and technical solutions was meant to reinforce the sense of the nation-state. As mentioned earlier, Nehru also believed that India occupied a privileged and implicitly hierarchical position, according to which the "sister continent" would benefit from her knowledge, training, and technology. Technoscientific cooperation provided India with "a new authority, a new moral stature, in the world" (Arnold 2013, 368).

Around the turn of the twenty-first century, however, India's model of cooperation was bound to change abruptly, with technoscientific cooperation becoming a medium for the acceleration of market expansion and global capital flows. As a result, almost half a century after his death, very little would remain of the sort of developmentalist and socialist ambitions cherished by Jawaharlal Nehru. Dreams of the nation endured, but the form taken by India's "gift to the world" would not be the same again. The next section examines this change.

Trade, Not Aid: A Defense of Indian Capitalism

The years 2003 and 2004 can be identified as a watershed moment for the resurgence of Indian cooperation in Africa and elsewhere. In the months leading up to President Kalam's announcement of PAN in 2004, the government of India—

a coalition led by the Bharatiya Janata Party (BJP), which had also supported Kalam's presidential candidacy—announced an important shift in the country's foreign policy. In his budget speech, the Indian minister of finance Jaswant Singh announced that India would no longer accept bilateral aid, with the exception of aid from five countries: the United States, the United Kingdom, Russia, Germany, and Japan (Six 2009). From then on, India would also no longer accept any tied aid whatsoever. The decision came just a few months after the government of India had decided to prepay US$3 billion of its external loans and repay its bilateral debt to all but four of its creditor states. The minister of finance further announced India's intention to cancel the debt of seven Heavily Indebted Poor Countries (HIPCs) and extend support, including grants and project assistance, to other developing countries (Ministry of Finance 2003, 20). As a result of the shift in policy, by the time PAN was launched in 2009, India had grown from being the world's largest recipient of foreign aid to being a global net donor (Katti, Chahoud, and Kaushik 2009). The factors underlying such a transition have been examined at length in media coverage, institutional reports, and academic literature. They include a rising preoccupation that some countries might use their donations to India as a foreign policy instrument as well as a sentiment that resorting to foreign aid was slowing down India's global ambitions, in particular her desire to obtain a permanent seat on the UN Security Council.[27] But beyond individual factors, these decisions were the expression of a resurgent sense of independence and strength. At stake was a broader attempt at defining a transnationally oriented national identity and presence—one that might disrupt still dominant West/non-West and North/South dichotomies.

Growing India-Africa trade has attracted significant attention in recent years. Plenty of news stories, policy notes, and financial reports have emphasized success stories and limitless economic opportunities.[28] While making no secret of the fact that India is drawn to Africa for its natural resources and access to markets, most of this writing—including academic writing—frames growing commercial relations between India and Africa as a win-win partnership. At the core of this equation, one finds the assumption according to which Indo-African trade comes with a special moral value: growing business is, in itself, considered a form of cooperation. While the Indian state openly acknowledges that its cooperation efforts are meant to foster business opportunities for its own, these are generally presented as being *desirable* for all. The distinction between trade and cooperation gets blurred, and it is precisely from this fuzzy zone of capital flows, state support, and a language of self-reliance and solidarity that Indo-African cooperation draws its originality.[29] In the words of Manmohan Singh, prime minister of India when PAN was launched, "Self-reliance means trade, not aid" (cited in Bhushan and Katyal 2004, 27).

"We believe that a new vision is required for Africa's development and participation in global affairs," Prime Minister Singh again noted during the Plenary session of the Second Africa-India Forum Summit, held in Addis Ababa in 2011 (M. Singh 2011). "We do not have all the answers, Singh explained, but we have some experience in nation building which we are happy to share with our African brothers and sisters" (M. Singh 2011).[30] The assistance Singh offered here was not of a metaphysical or moral kind, of the likes of vasudhaiva kutumbakam. Nor was it merely coarse trade. Rather, it presented Indian economic growth as a *model* to emulate. Using concepts such as capacity building, inclusive growth, and knowledge and technology transfer, cooperation with Africa contributes to asserting the legitimacy of an Indian model for economic growth. The notion of India becoming a role model for development and wealth creation is not new. Nor is it restricted to the African continent. As was suggested by Pankaj Mishra, it plays a key role in the self-fashioning of an Indian elite that has been expanding and entrenching itself in recent years (Mishra 2013). It can also be seen as a continuation of the kind of pedagogical politics practiced by Jawaharlal Nehru, via which India's contribution to global affairs also builds its status and ascendancy over other developing nations. As a senior official at the Ministry of External Affairs explained to me, "We know that aid is not working. What we propose is cooperation. We had the same problems here so we are in a good position to show them. We want them to understand how we developed!"[31]

By the time PAN was launched, South-South cooperation had little in common with earlier forms of Afro-Asian solidarity. Technoeconomic cooperation, as it was imagined by Jawaharlal Nehru in particular, was a modernist, socialist, and nation-building project. In sharp contrast, revamped versions of South-South cooperation are unabashedly capitalist: economic growth equates to development (Mawdsley 2011, 180). While the latter revolved around a collective understanding of freedom—national sovereignty—resurgent South-South cooperation aims at an economically integrated South with accelerated trade. To convey this shift in philosophy, ITEC hardly seemed like the right medium. This is when the Pan-African e-Network, announced in 2004 by Kalam, came into play. However, South-South cooperation remains a boundary-making technology in the sense that it enacts civilizational hierarchies while shaping the imagination of the nation. In continuance with a Nehruvian legacy, cooperation contributes to legitimizing India's global economic, cultural, and moral ascendancy.[32] In *Asia as Method*, Kuan-Hsing Chen warns that the downside of the postcolonial claiming of civilizational history may be that it falls into the logic of colonial competition "over which represents the Other of the West" (Chen 2010, 93). Claims to difference, Chen notes, may then reproduce the structure of ethnocentrism, and its imperialist cultural imaginary, by reasserting the centrality of the "opposed

West." In a project like PAN, South-South cooperation operated as a legitimation of a certain idea of India and its place in the world: its moral high ground, civilizational identity, and model for development, including for the distribution of medical care and expertise on a large scale. In order to examine this model, however, another story needs to be told. This is a fascinating story about the emergence of telemedicine in India. This is a story in which two distinct series of events mingled around the turn of the millennium, leading to the launch of PAN: the postcolonial development of space technology for "social good" and the rapid expansion of corporate hospitals across the country.

Space Technology for Development

When the Pan-African e-Network project was announced in 2004, the implementation of telemedicine networks in sub-Saharan Africa, and more widely in low- and middle-income countries, remained episodic and unusual.[33] Throughout the 1990s, a few transnational telemedicine networks had been implemented to facilitate the circulation of medical expertise to remote or underserved areas. These include humanitarian networks such as the HealthNet network, the Swinfen Charitable Trust, and the Réseau Afrique Francophone de Télémédecine (RAFT).[34] Transnational telemedicine experiments were also conducted by the US Department of Defense in US-Associated Pacific Islands (USAPI) and the National Aeronautics and Space Administration (NASA).[35] These early networks were aimed at the management of difficult patient cases, facilitating patient referral, and providing medical education. These were modest, low-cost pilot programs using store-and-forward technology and email communication systems. They also were primarily benevolent and experimental enterprises.[36] The genealogy of the Pan-African e-Network, however, is not to be located in Geneva or in Washington, DC. Rather, it can be traced back to the creation of the Indian Space Research Organisation (ISRO) and to its vision, according to which satellite technology should contribute to shaping India as a technologically modern and economically developed nation.

"There are some who question the relevance of space activities in a developing nation. To us, there is no ambiguity of purpose," Dr. Vikram Sarabhai said on February 2, 1968, in his speech during the dedication of the Thumba Equatorial Rocket Launch Station (TERLS) to the United Nations (cited in Harvey 2000, 129–30). "We do not have the fantasy of competing with the economically advanced nations in the explorations of the Moon or the planets or manned space flights," Sarabhai expressed, "but we are convinced that if we are to play a meaningful role nationally and in the community of nations, we must be second to none in the application of advanced technologies to the real problems of man and society which we find in this country" (cited in Harvey 2000, 129–30). The impact of space technology should be measured in economic and social terms, Sarabhai insisted. Vikram Sarabhai's vision for an indigenous space program in India was inspired by Prime Minister Nehru, who indeed placed science and technology at the center of the project of a modern India, free from the yoke of underdevelopment and dependence. For Nehru, it was through the development of scientific thought and technological mastery that the nation would find its way into the movement of universal history.[37] Science, development, and national unity were completely intertwined in his conception of the nation-state. It is in this spirit and still under the leadership of Nehru that the Department of Atomic Energy set up the Indian National Committee for Space Research (INCOSPAR) in 1962, with the explicit objective of studying the possibilities offered to India in the field of space research. Nehru appointed Sarabhai to head INCOSPAR. After a few years of developing sounding rocket technology within the framework of international cooperation programs, INCOSPAR became the Indian Space Research Organisation (ISRO) in 1969.

For scientific elites such as Sarabhai, whom Abdul Kalam would later consider a mentor, the development of an indigenous space program had to be a national priority on at least two grounds. First, space technology was to create long-term economic benefits, especially for the rural poor. As was suggested by the excerpt from his speech quoted earlier, Sarabhai believed it was essential for India to have a major space program in order to develop technology that could address the practical problems of the "common man" (*aam aadmi*). More than three decades before the concept took over the jargon of international institutions, he saw space technology as an opportunity to "leapfrog" stages of development.[38] This desire to develop programs based on their tangible applications in the lives of the greatest number of people is undoubtedly a distinctive feature of the history of the Indian space program. Secondly, for Sarabhai, ISRO was not simply to put existing technologies at the service of the Indian population. In collaboration with foreign partners, the aim was to develop indigenous space technology that would make India self-reliant and indeed a leader among the countries of the Third World.[39] ISRO's space program was to demonstrate how a newly independent state could harness science and technology to transform the existing social order. It would set an example, a *model* for others to follow.

On April 19, 1975, the first Indian-made satellite was launched into orbit. Named after the famous Indian astronomer and mathematician Aryabhata (476–550 CE), the satellite was launched by a Soviet rocket with the objective, among others, of studying stellar rays, solar neutrons, and gamma radiation from solar flares. One of the many experiments carried out by Aryabhata was the transmission of electrocardiogram (ECG) signals. As a paper published by a scientist from ISRO suggested, "The results were quite encouraging and demonstrated the feasibility of extending medical help to remote areas through the use of satellites" (Rao 1978, 127). Thus, as early as 1975, ISRO was conducting its first telemedicine experiment. However, it would take two more decades before telemedicine came to the forefront of ISRO's social mission.

In the meantime, ISRO's developmentalist and social mission expanded in other directions.[40] A flagship illustration of this mission is the Satellite Instructional Television Experiment (SITE), launched in 1975 as an ambitious attempt to harness satellite technology for educational purposes in rural India. But while Aryabhata was the result of a collaboration with the Soviet Union, SITE was the result of an agreement signed in 1969 between Vikram Sarabhai and NASA.[41] Sarabhai's idea was to test the effectiveness of television as a communication medium for popular education and rural development. Six years later, with Satish Dhawan now at the helm of ISRO—Sarabhai passed in 1971—NASA moved its ATS-6 communications satellite over India. For a year or so, SITE broadcast a range of television programs covering topics such as agriculture, health, hygiene, and family planning in over 2,400 Indian villages. SITE was the first attempt to deliver educational programs directly to rural areas. Eminent science fiction writer Sir Arthur C. Clarke, who was a consultant on the project, called SITE the "greatest communications experiment in history" (Clarke 2004, iii).

On the face of it, SITE confirmed Sarabhai's vision: satellite technology could be used for national development, and there was a demand for such programs. However, the literature that retrospectively assessed SITE also insisted on the limitations of a top-down, state-developmentalist paradigm, which remained too distant from the actual lifeworlds in the villages where the programs were broadcast. Anthropologist William Mazzarella suggests that the debates surrounding the deployment of SITE were marked by a dynamic of "close distance"—namely, "the pursuit of a kind of programming content that would at once be 'close' enough to resonate with the existing concrete lifeways of audiences and 'distant' enough to prompt a desire for progress, as understood within the discourse of development" (Mazzarella 2012, 227). As it aimed to integrate the underprivileged in the national development effort, SITE staged a tension between the dream of a decentralized leapfrogging of established social hierarchies on the one hand and the enduring promise of a centralized, unifying movement of integration on the other. With its capacity to reach remote locations and peoples, the satellite materialized the tension, constitutive of the postmodern nation, between *national unification* (making India present to itself through communication and education) and *distant connections* (including relationships with the country's sociocultural diversity and economic disparity). As historian Asif Siddiqi suggests, although there is an inclusive imperative at play ("disseminate information to the masses"), India's dreams of a television broadcasting satellite to educate the country's poor also "betrays a paternalistic and *exclusive* view of the future of India. . . . Actual people are absent here except in the metonym of an undifferentiated whole—'the masses,' the local" (Siddiqi 2015, 46). This production of distance via connectivity would remain a key feature of ISRO's developmentalist mission, including its telemedicine program in the decades that followed. And indeed, as we should later see, of the Pan-African e-Network.

In the years that followed the SITE experiment, which remained to a large extent dependent on foreign technology, ISRO worked hard on developing an indigenous communications satellite infrastructure. On June 19, 1981, ISRO launched India's first communications satellite, the Ariane Passenger PayLoad Experiment (APPLE), from the Guiana Space Center, a French launch base near Kourou in French Guiana. Two years later, the Indian National Satellite System (INSAT) was set up. INSAT is a series of satellites in geostationary orbit aimed at supporting the country's telecommunications needs, among other things. After a few years of using foreign-built satellites, ISRO launched Insat 2A in 1992, the first telecommunications satellite to be built entirely in India, albeit using foreign launchers. Then, in 2001, ISRO used the Geosynchronous Satellite Launch Vehicle (GSLV) for the first time, which would allow it to launch its own satellites into geostationary orbit. By the time PAN was implemented in 2009, ISRO had successfully launched twenty-one communications satellites, making it the largest national communications system in the Asia-Pacific region.

This achievement can be seen as a material manifestation of Nehru and Sarabhai's early nation-building aspirations and visions. Although it was not always evident *how* Indian space science would practically benefit other developing nations, its power always seemed to reside in its capacity to fuel the imagination for other science and technology futures, rejecting the approach taken by global superpowers. This power of demonstration, or modeling, was also always inseparable from the kind of pedagogical performance of politics already staged at Bandung and by which the nation established itself as an example to follow.

Politics of Care

"I think it is a very wonderful contribution to the healthcare of the people who live in rural villages and I hope that people all over the world will follow your lead, because if they do then the benefits of the hi-tech medicine can go to everyone and not just people who live in big cities" (cited in Warrier 2000). It is with these words that on March 24, 2000, US president Bill Clinton inaugurated the first site of what would become the largest telemedicine network in India—and one of the largest in the world. Clinton was on an official visit to Apollo Hospital in Hyderabad, one of two hospitals (the other being in Chennai) chosen to provide teleconsultations to a hospital in the village of Aragonda in Andhra Pradesh. The home village of Dr. Prathap Reddy, founder of Apollo Hospitals—the first corporate chain of hospitals in India—Aragonda was to have unique access to medical expertise. Not only had Apollo opened a modern hospital there with primary and secondary care services two years earlier, but it was now connected to two of the country's most recognized hospitals as part of a pilot project set up by ISRO and Apollo Hospitals. When we met in Chennai many years later, the director of the Apollo Telemedicine Networking Foundation (ATNF) Dr. K. Ganapathy recalled the events leading to the pilot in these terms:

> In 1999, luckily at the same time, the ISRO, they were also looking at societal implications to use satellite technology. They would not get funding in a country like India, for high-class based technology unless it has some relevance! They were looking out for applications that would be of benefit for the man on the street, so that the Parliament would increase the funding of the space agency. You must understand that was 1997–1998. India now is totally different. So then they realized that providing healthcare to rural areas is a fantastic way of using satellite technology. It was already being used in the field of education. We approached them for healthcare. The climate was just right. We did not have to spend too much time convincing them. They were happy to cooperate with us.[42]

Over the next four years, nearly 4,000 teleconsultations were apparently conducted from Aragonda. After only a few months, ISRO proceeded to expand the network. Other hospital chains wanted to join in.[43] States inquired about the availability of services, requesting that their local district hospitals join the network. By 2008, ISRO's telemedicine network connected 400 sites: over 350 district hospitals (offering primary and secondary care services) were connected to some 40 tertiary care hospitals belonging to different hospital chains.[44] ISRO's network most often connects private tertiary care hospitals located in metropolitan areas such as Chennai, New Delhi, and Bangalore to public district hospitals located in suburban or rural areas. Over these few years, more than 400,000 teleconsultations reportedly took place through the network.

Because of its social mission, ISRO does not rent the bandwidth used for telemedicine to hospitals. Rather, when ISRO agrees to connect a hospital to the network, it provides the satellite and IT equipment free of charge. Connected district hospitals are provided with some IT equipment—for example, a personal computer, medical software for sharing patient data, and a few diagnostic instruments such as an ECG, an X-ray machine, and an X-ray. In exchange for free satellite connectivity, ISRO requires that teleconsultations are offered free of cost by participating tertiary hospitals.[45] But in spite of this social mission, ISRO's telemedicine network has from the beginning been structured as a public-private partnership (PPP).[46] As a government agency, ISRO was to act as a facilitator of care, serving as a technical and logistical intermediary between the patient, his or her physician, and a corporate tertiary care hospital.[47]

To fully assess the role played by ISRO's telemedicine in India, it is important to understand that ISRO's network emerged in the context of and indeed contributed to the rapid emergence of corporate tertiary care hospitals in India. When Apollo Hospitals opened its first hospital in 1983 in Chennai, it was the first Indian hospital operated by a publicly traded company. At the time, hospitals were run by charities or the state. Over the course of this research, I have heard many versions of the "Apollo story." This is a quasi-mythological story featuring Dr. Prathap Reddy as a pioneer fighting before its time against the countless bureaucratic pitfalls of a commercially inward-looking India. According to the story, it took several meetings with influential politicians to convince them to let him borrow from banks: hospitals did not usually qualify for such loans at the time. American colleagues had to invest. Importing equipment was difficult, if not impossible. However, the situation was about to change. Gradually, during the 1980s, some timid reforms opened the door to a greater role for the private sector. As early as 1983, the National Health Policy proposed to expand the supply of health services through the use of the private sector (Thomas and Krishnan 2010). Then came the 1991 economic reforms. As in other sectors of the Indian economy, these would have a major impact. The measures that were put in place included major cuts in state investment in health, a wide opening to private investment, and the introduction of user fees.[48]

The reforms set the table for the rapid growth of the corporate hospital industry in India. In the 1990s and 2000s, chains such as Apollo Hospitals, Fortis Healthcare, and Narayana Hrudayalaya expanded their operations at a phenomenal rate. By the time PAN was launched in 2009, Apollo Hospitals had gone from a single hospital in 1983 to operating over 40 hospitals, with a capacity of nearly 9,000 beds, in India alone. For its part, the Narayana Hrudayalaya Group—now renamed Narayana Health—operated fourteen hospitals with more than five thousand beds. Fortis Healthcare, which was set up in 2001, was challenging Apollo for the title of national leader with some sixty hospitals in India. Hundreds of other private hospitals, the majority of which were owned by a dozen companies, grew across the country, almost exclusively in urban areas. Nearly thirty years after the first Apollo hospital opened, the Indian health care market was valued at more than US$30 billion and growing at more than 30 percent per year (India Africa Connect 2012). By the time PAN was launched, a vast majority of hospital beds were in the private sector (Mahal, Debroy, and Bandhari 2010).

The economic reforms, and the emergence of corporate hospitals in the 1990s and 2000s, did not only reconfigure the modalities of health care provision. They transformed the politics of care in India, including the role of the state and of public health care infrastructure. The health sector reform put emphasis on efficiency, efficacy, and quality of health care services. But this was soon interpreted as an expanded role for markets (Kumar 2009, 19). The structural adjustment program undertaken with the reforms put great pressure on the Indian state to invest less and less in the hospital sector. The state did not entirely withdraw from the scene: while it abandoned its role as a public supplier of hospital services, it also actively supported the growth of corporate hospital chains. A host of financial provisions favorable to private investment were introduced, and corporate hospitals were awarded subsidies, urban land, and tax exemptions. In other words, the Indian state sought to reinvent its public mission from providing hospital care to funding and regulating the private sector. Major hospital chains were the main beneficiaries of these new orientations (Lefebvre 2010, 10). The expansion of corporate hospitals was often supported by public-private partnerships (PPP) in which the state would provide infrastructure in exchange for which hospitals would have to treat some patients free of cost. For example, the government would provide land at no cost and contribute financially to the construction of a hospital while in return the hospital would agree to use a certain percentage of its beds for the free treatment of poor patients.[49]

The model taken by ISRO's telemedicine network is therefore part of a wider politics of care in which the Indian state reimagined its role as a health care facilitator instead of a care provider. Telemedicine expanded in India as a PPP. It concurred with massive disinvestment in public health infrastructures, particularly affecting remote and rural areas. While ISRO provided the satellite infrastructure free of cost, rapidly growing hospital chains could reach new patient populations across the country. In telemedicine, the state does not provide health care. Rather, it subsidizes the satellite infrastructure aimed at building access.

Like ISRO's telemedicine network in India, the Pan-African e-Network was launched with the aim to reach new patients. However, PAN did not solely export medical care. It exemplified a politics of care that was experimentally developed in India. As a scientist who was in charge of ISRO's telemedicine program for many years pointed out to me, "The Indian telemedicine program should be a very good example for developing countries."[50] What was being extended was not merely a physical network. It was a politics of care, which was also a model for market creation and economic growth. In the years preceding the launch of PAN, then, telemedicine accelerated the privatization of hospital care in India. Just like with

South-South cooperation—remember Prime Minister Singh: "self-reliance means trade, not aid"—there was a shift from state-centric developmentalism toward a model in which the state became a medium for capital and market opportunities. While both models shared a belief in the power of science and technology to shape the nation, the modalities of intervention had very little in common.

Distance and Disparity

By the turn of the millennium, demographic data clearly indicated that the health indices of the rural population in India were much worse than those of the urban population. The second round of the National Family Health Survey (1997–98), for example, revealed that health inequalities between urban and rural areas were worsening (International Institute for Population Sciences (IIPS) and ORC Macro 2000). The report noted that the rural mortality rates were considerably higher than in urban areas, including maternal, infant, and child mortality rates, which were almost two times higher in rural areas. The prevalence of conditions such as tuberculosis, malaria, and asthma was also found to be considerably higher in rural areas. Over the following years, research underlined the factors explaining this situation: inadequate public expenditure on health, imbalance in resource allocation (including among states), and a greater proportion of resources being directed toward urban-based and curative services (Balarajan, Selvaraj, and Subramanian 2011). By the turn of the millennium, it had become evident that the unregulated privatization of the health care sector, accompanied by stagnating public health expenditures, had made health care less affordable and less accessible for the poor, more so in rural areas (Sen 2001).

Health care inequity was a complex socioeconomic problem reflecting wider inequalities as well as the result of an underfunded public health care system. However, one factor in particular was often identified as the main culprit for the inequity between urban and rural areas: the lack of physical access to curative health services in rural areas. The National Health Profile (NHP) of India, for example, showed that the number of beds in government hospitals in urban areas was more than twice that in rural areas (CBHI 2008). The rapid development of the private sector in urban areas had resulted in an unplanned and unequal geographical distribution of services (Balarajan, Selvaraj, and Subramanian 2011). While almost three-quarters of the Indian population lived in rural areas, a vast majority of the hospitals, doctors, and paraprofessionals were located in urban areas. Throughout the 2000s, it became clear that corporate hospital chains were failing to reach populations outside the urban centers. Put simply, opening hospitals in rural areas does not fit into their business model: while there is a demand for hospital services in rural areas, it is not concentrated enough. Hospital chains are primarily attracted to areas with a large pool of potential patients.[51] This is not the case in rural India, given that the cost of treatment in corporate hospitals is prohibitively high for a majority of the population. Hence, as the state's role shifted from being a provider of hospital care to merely facilitating the private sector's expansion, the divide between rural and urban access to health care widened.

It is under these circumstances that telemedicine came to be seen as *the* appropriate technology to build access to and reach rural and remote populations. The Tenth Five Year Plan of the Planning Commission of India is a remarkable document in that regard. Approved in 2002, at a moment when telemedicine started to expand, the Tenth Plan recognized that the health system suffered "from inequitable distribution of institutions and manpower" (Planning Commission 2002b, 82). Even though every year the country produces over seventeen thousand doctors in medicine, the plan noted, "There are huge gaps in critical manpower in institutions providing primary healthcare, especially in the remote rural and tribal areas where healthcare needs are the greatest" (Planning Commission 2002b, 82). In response to the "poor functional status of the system" in rural areas, the plan did not suggest raising public investment in the primary health care infrastructure. Rather, in order to properly reach this underserved population, the plan suggested, services would have to be "restructured": they would have to be better *integrated*. A key focus of the plan was therefore to "build up an integrated health system with appropriate screening, regulating access at different levels and efficient referral linkages" (Planning Commission 2002b, 82). Mentioned over seventy times in the health section of the plan, the notion of "integration" condensed much of the proposed vision. Central to integration was the establishment of appropriate referral linkages between primary, secondary, and tertiary care levels. This was to be done—and this is identified as the second area of focus of the plan—via the "development of appropriate two-way referral systems utilizing information technology (IT) tools to improve communication, consultation and referral right from primary care to tertiary" (Planning Commission 2002b, 83).

The Tenth Plan, therefore, framed health care inequity as a technical issue of geographical access. Telemedicine appeared to be the appropriate technology to solve this issue.[52] Telemedicine in India was never aimed at repairing a broken public health care system but rather at circumventing some of the most blatant challenges it is facing. With health care access being increasingly fragmented and unevenly distributed, satellite technology promised to integrate primary health centers (PHCs) and district hospitals inside tertiary care pathways. Care units accessible in rural areas would be hierarchically nested into a nationwide network of corporate tertiary care hospitals. As mentioned in the introduction to this book, telemedicine promises to vertically integrate the medical facility of the country. In this networked, vertically integrated health infrastructure, corporate chains have no need to open hospitals in rural areas: knowledge and patients are accessible at a distance. For corporate hospitals, telemedicine does not simply respond to preexisting patient populations. It produces new remote patient populations disentangled from the state as a care provider. Telemedicine in India was designed to be the gift that keeps on *taking*. So was the Pan-African e-Network.

Modeling Growth

Telemedicine in India, I have suggested so far, has transformed ISRO's social mission into a nationwide satellite infrastructure driving the market expansion of corporate hospitals. The deployment of telemedicine in India as a public-private partnership has little in common with the type of nation-building that presided over the creation of ISRO. There is a clear break with a Nehruvian approach for which nation-building is tied to socioeconomic self-determination and a strong state presence. By contrast, the expansion of telemedicine in India blurs the distinction between social and economic development. However, what is common to ISRO's original developmentalist mission and its entrepreneurial experiment with telemedicine is that in both cases, satellite technology is a site of affective and imaginative investment. In either case, the satellite is both a performance and a mode of rule that constitutes relations between the state and citizens. Satellite communication seeds the imagination of *future* economic growth—in the name of the nation.

The Pan-African e-Network embodied such a desire for connectivity and growth. However, the history of PAN is not simply about boosting but also about *modeling* growth: giving it direction, setting an example, and imposing order. South-South cooperation always was a boundary-making technology (Abraham 2014, 3). So was telemedicine in India. Transnational flows cannot be assumed to be the "basic infrastructural fact" (Harvey, Jensen, and Morita 2016) of a project like PAN. The history of PAN here stands in contrast with widespread narratives of global health that, as mentioned earlier, tend to emphasize the unmooring of health issues from both nation and state. For sure, telemedicine in India shares global health's commitment to market-based, technological solutions to complex health phenomena. However, the history of PAN brings the nation back in full force. For Abdul Kalam, among other PAN stakeholders, visions of economic growth are indissociable from dreams of the nation. Dreams of the nation, in turn, have as much to do with reverting to an idealized past as with embracing an open-ended future. They stage an ancient cultural identity, a unique "gift to the world" whose renaissance has been too long in coming.[53]

As years of scholarship on design and technology have shown, we need to take seriously the dreams, metaphors, and visions that shape the way designers frame their projects' relationships to the world. And yet as work on infrastructure has taught us, infrastructure is never a given: it is a relational, dynamic sociotechnical formation that emerges *in practice*, even if it is contingent on social structures. Similarly, as the next few chapters will make clear, the Pan-African e-Network was not a stable object. It was elusive, as opaque as it was spectacular, and its actual effects were hard to predict. Whether it be its designers, its implementers or sponsors, or the hospitals' corporate managers, we should not expect that any of the agents involved in PAN held the power to enforce linear development (Harvey, Jensen, and Morita 2016). PAN did not function according to the plans of anyone in particular, nor did it simply materialize specific ideas or interests. PAN aimed to give form and model emergent relations, and this ambition came with all kinds of practical consequences. However, technical assemblages do not easily become models themselves. A key question is how an excessive project such as PAN, which was not particularly effective from a strictly economic point of view (it produced little commercial value on its own), was recuperated and "put to work" on different levels.

A key challenge in this book is therefore to describe how PAN's relations unfolded on the ground instead of assuming that they simply extended historically dominant forms of boundary making. How could these relations, in PAN, open onto new imaginative possibilities? Can the mobilization of the past leave new horizons open, pointing toward and nourishing a fascination for the future? Is there, for example, a spirit left from Bandung that could produce new forms of nonalignment rather than the mere reiteration of past dreams and promises?

MEDICINE FROM THE AIR

**Connectivity is strength. Connectivity is wealth.
Connectivity is progress.**

—Dr. A. P. J. Abdul Kalam (2007, 172)

Omar had been admitted a few weeks earlier to the pediatric cardiology department of the CHNU Fann in Dakar. The four-year-old boy presented respiratory distress with vomiting and abdominal pain. Omar was hospitalized with ascites. When cardiologists performed an electrocardiogram, they realized he had a complete atrioventricular block, a defect in the transmission of electrical impulses between the atria and ventricles of the heart. His heart was beating too slowly, not perfusing the organs sufficiently and not receiving enough blood to function properly. The treating doctors at CHNU Fann were unanimous: Omar needed a pacemaker. But things were not simple. There are two types of pacemakers. First, there is the transvenous pacemaker, installed via an endocavitary venous route. Under local anesthesia, the pacemaker is installed by the cardiologist, who makes an incision near the collarbone, introduces the electrodes and the pacemaker, and then pushes the electrodes to the heart. This is a minor operation that is regularly performed in CHNU Fann's cardiology department.

In other cases, however, it is necessary to open the thorax to put the electrodes in place on the surface of the myocardium. This is called an epicardial pacemaker. The procedure to install that pacemaker is more complex, and it must be performed by a surgeon. Cardiologists at Fann debated Omar's case because a decision had to be made regarding the type of pacemaker that would be the most appropriate for a child his age. The cardiology team at Fann had never installed a pacemaker in such a young child. Also, a pacemaker is expensive. Since it has to be replaced every five to seven years, it represents a significant financial burden for the family. Omar's family did not have health insurance, so they would have to cover all of the costs themselves. Furthermore, this is an irreversible decision: once the pacemaker is installed, the patient becomes dependent on it. For all of these reasons, some cardiologists thought it might be better to wait until Omar was older. Many questions remained: Should they do it now or wait? Would the patient need to be referred to surgery, or could the procedure be done in cardiology? The cardiologists agreed on at least one thing: this was an atypical case, and it would be a good idea to seek an external opinion. Booking an appointment with "the Indians" seemed like the obvious solution.

A few days later, a teleconsultation took place. TCIL engineers at CHNU Fann had difficulty getting an appointment with a cardiologist at Apollo Hospital, so the teleconsultation was with Dr. Chopra from Fortis Escorts Heart Institute in New Delhi. Dr. Chopra is a senior pediatric cardiologist who has practiced in many countries. Before the teleconsultation, he consulted the patient's medical file and reviewed the results of the electrocardiogram. Also present during the teleconsultation were the TCIL engineers from both hospitals involved as well as Dr. Wade, Omar's treating physician at Fann, and Dr. Leye. The session lasted about twenty minutes. Various issues were discussed. First, the doctors at Fann wanted to hear from their Indian colleagues about the need for a pacemaker and the urgency of the situation. Dr. Chopra's opinion was unambiguous: Omar needed to have the pacemaker installed as soon as possible. Then Dr. Leye wanted to know what type of pacemaker was appropriate for such a young child. The discussion rapidly turned to the general approach to the surgery. According to Dr. Chopra, if certain precautions were taken, it would be possible to insert the pacemaker through a vein. Following the teleconsultation, the cardiologists at Fann decided to transfer Omar's case to the Department of Thoracic and Cardiovascular Surgery (DTCS). A few weeks later, Omar was successfully operated on. He did not have to be referred elsewhere, neither for a second opinion nor for surgery.

Telemedicine, I was often told by its users, allowed clinicians to take a step back and get some distance from a patient's case. It could make up for deficits, and most specifically for a lack of perspective, expressed in terms of distance.[1] Another spatial metaphor that was used by some PAN users to describe its impact refers to the network as "opening up the clinic." Network infrastructure made the room bigger.[2] This movement of opening, however, was not spontaneous. It shared little in common with popular imaginaries of networks as tools for global circulation and extension. As examined in chapter 1, PAN carried the promise to carve out new digital South-South routes for the making of global biomedicine. PAN was a big, flamboyant gift rooted in situated transnational histories. Connecting more than fifty hospitals, it was a private network designed as a public-private partnership (PPP): funded by the Indian state and with products and services provided by Indian companies including corporate hospitals, computer and medical equipment vendors, and telecom corporations. PAN was a unique market opportunity. The cartography of a project like PAN, however, entails directing the same attention to the properties of its material infrastructure as it does to the "dynamics of world history and the forces of capitalism" (Harvey, Krohn-Hansen, and Nustad 2019, 8–9).

In this chapter, I examine the materialities and practices that enacted the network as a medium for exchange of expertise and the practice of medicine. The chapter suggests that medicine in PAN was primarily shaped by nonclinical spaces, infrastructures, and labor. It does so by attending to the power of materials, cared for and mediated by human labor, that forged clinical and market relations in PAN. First, there is the material and historical specificities of network infrastructure. PAN was built out of a combination of a fiber-optic network, a submarine cable system, and satellite technology—all of which were operated and maintained for over a decade. It was imagined as a large, scalable entity that would create immediate, traceable trajectories between India and Africa. However, I suggest that infrastructure in PAN never was finite or stable. In dialogue with the work of Susan Leigh Star on infrastructure, this chapter challenges "connectionist" imaginations of network infrastructure, which emphasize circulation and extension over space. Rather, the chapter insists on the embeddedness of digital medicine and the enduring importance of the places connected by and composing PAN. The chapter documents the routines and slow-paced operations that sustained the spatial order of the clinic in PAN. Particular attention is given to the administrative and technical work carried out by the network engineers who supported the network's everyday medical activities.[3] PAN engineers held PAN together by mediating among hospital environments, technology, and medical practitioners. By paying attention to the entanglement of human labor and the sheer materiality of network infrastructure, the chapter shows how people and things were working together to enact digital medicine, thus also challenging human-centric understandings of knowledge and care at a distance.

Peoples and Places

Established in 1955, the Centre Hospitalier National Universitaire (CHNU) of Fann covers an area of one hundred acres in the southwestern part of the Senegalese capital, in the center of the Fann Residence district. Neighboring Cheikh Anta Diop University (the country's largest university campus), CHNU Fann is a public university hospital that combines training, tertiary care, and medical research. With more than three hundred beds, Fann serves patients from all over Senegal. To some extent, the institution is also a regional center of expertise to which physicians and patients travel from neighboring countries to receive training or treatment. Fann Hospital, in other words, is a respected institution with a good reputation and status.

The Pan-African e-Network was in operation at Fann between 2009 and 2018. The studios of PAN were located on the top floor of a large building located near the entrance of Fann, on Cheikh Anta Diop Avenue. They occupied the main room of a floor entirely dedicated to Fann's telemedicine activities. While PAN was arguably the most prominent telemedicine network at Fann, it was not the only one. A few meters away from PAN's studios, for instance, was a room hosting a team of engineers employed by the hospital to launch a pilot project aimed at connecting Fann to regional health centers in Senegal. Two or three workers, sometimes more, worked from the room. PAN's offices were located at the other end of the corridor, in a large room mainly dedicated to the network's activities. On occasion, the room also served as a multipurpose room, for example hosting small conferences or seminars.

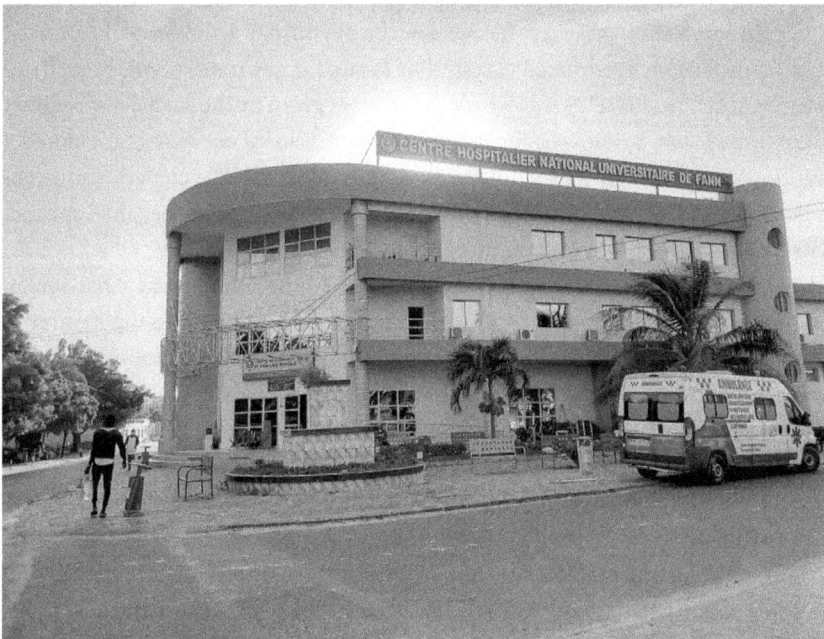

FIGURE 1. Building hosting the PAN studios at CHNU Fann in Dakar. Photo by author.

Two engineers worked full time on the network at CHNU Fann. Employed by TCIL, Jean-Louis and Sada spent most of their days at their respective workstations within PAN's studios. Both Senegal citizens, a rare situation in PAN given that TCIL engineers were generally dispatched from India, Jean-Louis and Sada were graduate students in software engineering at the National Institute of Information Technology (NIIT) in Dakar. In the middle of the room stood the main workstation, furnished with a microscope, a laser printer, and three computers, all equipped with microphones and cameras. Next to the workstation, rows of chairs were set up facing a wall where continuing medical education (CME) sessions were projected every day. Then, there was a studio and a server room. The studio was home to the teleconsultations while the server room, a relatively small room with clear glass walls, contained the servers required for PAN's activities.

PAN studios in Indian hospitals were usually divided into three or four different rooms. The case of Apollo Hospital is fairly representative. When arriving on-site, you would walk through the Production Control Room. As the name suggests, this room was used to oversee the production of teleconsultation and CME sessions. It housed several computers as well as a digital production switcher to adjust the sound and image quality of the CME sessions. At Apollo, this room was the workstation of Ashoka, TCIL's engineer on-site. Like his colleagues elsewhere in India, this was where he oversaw the day-to-day activities of the project. The control room overlooked two studios located in separate rooms. First, there was the CME studio. This was where the courses given by the medical specialists were filmed. The studio was furnished with professional equipment including a lighting system and a high-definition camera on a tripod. The camera pointed to a desk, behind which sat the doctor who had come to deliver the CME session. On the desk, there was a computer screen on which the speaker could see his or her PowerPoint presentation scrolling. Next to the camera was a flat-screen television displaying images of the doctors or trainees attending the session in the African sites—or images of empty chairs. Then, the control room was adjacent to the telemedicine studio. The room consisted of a workstation with a few chairs, a computer, speakers, headphones, and a seventeen-inch flat-screen with a webcam. This was where the doctor and the TCIL engineer would sit during teleconsultations. Behind the telemedicine studio was the server room, which, like at Fann, housed servers, modems, and routers in two large towers.

After graduating in 2005, Dr. Leye left Senegal for three years of postdoctoral training at a pediatric hospital in the Paris area. The pediatric cardiologist in his thirties came back to Senegal in 2008 and started to practice at the Department of Cardiology at CHNU Fann. A few months later, PAN was launched. Dr. Leye remembers having been approached by the head of his department, inquiring about his interest in acting as a "delegate" for Fann cardiologists who might want

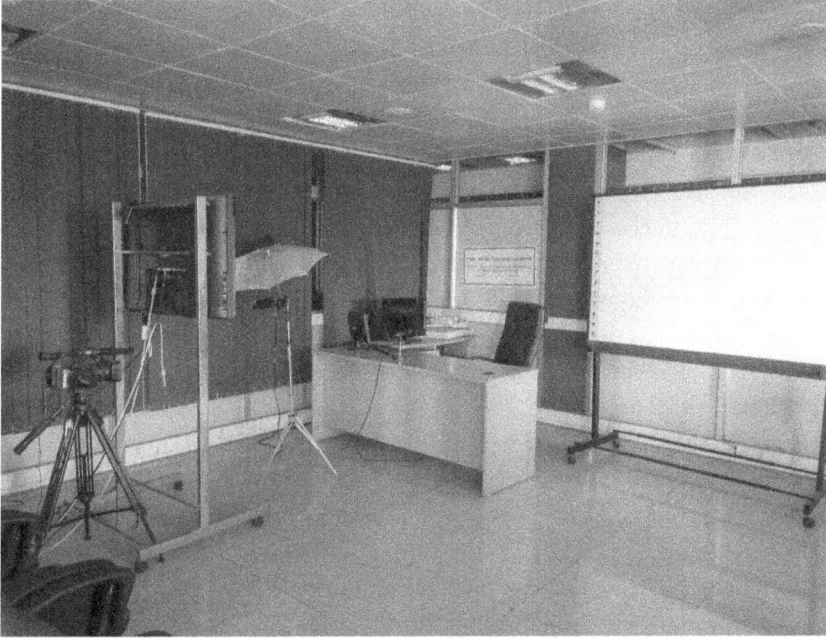

FIGURE 2. A CME studio of the Pan-African e-Network in an Indian hospital. Photo by author.

to use PAN—an assignment he readily accepted. Dr. Leye's main duties were to connect with Indian specialists to present cases of patients from his department. The patients were sometimes his own but not always. Dr. Leye explains, "The cases that are presented to the Indians, we discuss them first among ourselves. . . . Then we share our experience with people [Indian doctors] who sometimes have more experience in certain fields."[4]

Every week, Dr. Leye thus walked into the PAN studio at CHNU Fann. Dr. Leye used PAN to get third-party opinions on patient cases discussed during the cardiology staff meetings, or "staffs," which are held every Friday. A staff is a meeting where physicians gather to discuss certain cases, usually of hospitalized patients. PAN was used to get additional qualified opinions on cases that were still considered problematic, or nonconsensual, after a staff meeting. The cases examined through PAN often dealt with pediatric surgery, a field in which cardiologists at Fann have little experience: "On the one hand, there is a scientific exchange. Every time we do a tele-expertise [with PAN], there is a scientific exchange. Either because we have a doubt about the diagnosis and we want a specialist to give us a confirmation, or we have made the diagnosis, but in terms of surgery, we have no experience. So we want to ask the opinion of someone who has been confronted with this type of situation on several occasions. From that point of view, there is a scientific benefit for us. On the other hand, there is also a benefit for the patient. Because when they give us their opinion, it allows us to readjust our management of the patient."[5]

The Department of Neurology at Fann was another frequent user of the network. The neurologist delegated to PAN was Dr. Sow. Completing the third year of a four-year internship, Dr. Sow was informed of the existence of PAN by the head of his department, Dr. Faye, who sometimes used the network himself. Dr. Sow was mainly chosen to act as a delegate because of his English-speaking skills. As with cardiology, the cases referred to PAN were discussed beforehand during a staff meeting. Every week, neurologists selected a case, prepared a summary, and brought it along with images to PAN's engineers. Then, on Thursday mornings, generally on a fixed schedule, there was a teleconsultation. A Fann neurologist would present the case to the Indian colleagues, and Dr. Sow helped with the translation. The neurologists' reasons for using PAN were similar to the cardiologists'—namely, a mix of scientific interest and support in the management of patients for whom an outside opinion could prove useful. According to Dr. Faye, PAN brought a "new vision" to problematic cases: "Sometimes, if we have difficulties on the diagnostic level, we want them to suggest something else so that we have a new vision."[6] Dr. Sow, however, suggests that sometimes teleconsultations were requested out of scientific interest but without any potential benefit for patient treatment: "It can be simply for scientific interest, it means that it's not necessarily for the patient. Because there are many conditions in neurology for which nothing can be done. So sometimes it's just to know that when he has these symptoms, well this could be it. It could be patients who have passed away. So, frankly, it's not for the patient anymore, it's for the doctors, it's so that we know that if we have the same case again, we should think about what. . . . But very often, it is when we're having difficulties either with the diagnosis or with the treatment."[7]

The medical specialties involved in PAN were diverse. They included radiology, gastroenterology, dermatology, urology, ophthalmology, oncology, plastic surgery, and pathology.[8] The types of cases referred to the network were no less varied and included rare conditions such as Ebstein's anomaly, Marfan syndrome, and cauda equina syndrome but also much more common conditions such as tetralogy of Fallot, multiple myeloma, and chronic constipation.[9] Usually, there was only one teleconsultation at a time. Teleconsultations were used primarily, but not exclusively, to discuss the cases of inpatients. Sometimes they took place on an emergency basis, but most often there were at least twenty-four hours between the request for a teleconsultation and the actual teleconsultation. As mentioned previously, the cases presented on the network were often problematic, rare, or complex for one reason or another. At CHNU Fann, they most often involved reaching out to an Indian cardiologist, cardiac surgeon, neurologist, or neurosurgeon. For example, when PAN was launched, pediatric expertise was in full development at Fann, and cardiologists did not have much experience with pediatric surgery.[10]

Although this was not standardized, most teleconsultations lasted about half an hour. They were always conducted in English. Patients were rarely present although they may have, on occasion, accompanied the treating physician to a teleconsultation. Doctors at Fann did not always connect with Apollo Hospital; they sometimes consulted colleagues from other Indian hospitals—for instance, from the All India Institute of Medical Sciences (AIIMS) in New Delhi. In addition to CHNU Fann, other major users of the network included Victoria Hospital (Mahé, Seychelles), SSR National Hospital (Pamplemousses, Mauritius), Lagos University Teaching Hospital (Lagos, Nigeria), Bosaso General Hospital (Bosaso, Somalia), and Black Lion Hospital (Addis Ababa, Ethiopia). Other hospitals barely used the network if at all.

Hospitals connected to the Pan-African e-Network were not interchangeable, generic sites through which universal knowledge would circulate. Biomedical practices and the availability of prescription drugs and diagnostic testing, for example, could vary greatly among connected hospitals. As is illustrated by the case of Mamadou, discussed below, it was not uncommon for the recommended diagnostic tests or treatment to be unavailable locally. Sometimes the teleconsultation would lead to a patient being transferred to another hospital, city, or country, whether it be in Africa, Europe, or India. The making of global biomedicine in PAN entailed a constant mediation between disparate medical worlds. It was always contingent on improvisations and dislocations of many kinds, in which older places and routes would often end up playing much more important roles than might have been expected.

A Global Clinic

In the manner he greeted Ashoka, it was obvious that Dr. Ambedkar was not visiting the premises of the Pan-African e-Network for the first time. After exchanging a few words with the TCIL engineer, he walked rapidly toward the telemedicine studio. In his early forties, Dr. Ambedkar is a pediatric cardiologist at Apollo Children's Hospital in Chennai. At the moment PAN was launched, he had just moved back to India. After completing his medical training at Madras Medical College, Dr. Ambedkar did like many other Indian medical specialists: he left the country for most of a decade, to train and work in the United Kingdom. He came back to Chennai with an opportunity to practice in one of the best pediatric hospitals in the country, a stone's throw away from Apollo Hospital's main building.

It was a little past 4:00 p.m., and Dr. Ambedkar had just finished his regular shift. Even though PAN's studios were not far from the hospital, he preferred to book his appointments for teleconsultations at the end of the day, thus avoiding losing too much time traveling between sites. As he sat down in the telemedicine studio, Dr. Ambedkar was followed by Ashoka. A medical file was already displayed on the computer screen. The file consisted of a two-page Word document starting with a general presentation of the patient: age, complaints, and symptoms. The patient's medical history was summarized in a single sentence: "History of dyspnea and squatting until primary infancy." This was followed by the patient's heart rate and percentage of percutaneous saturation. Then, a section described the examinations carried out on the patient and included the primary results. Finally, the document presented the diagnostic impressions of the treating physician: "Irregular form of tetralogy of Fallot with hypoplasia of left pulmonary artery and partial anomaly of left pulmonary venous return." Then, at the bottom of the document, two questions stood out in large red characters: "What do you think about this diagnosis? What can we do for this boy? What kind of surgery and how?"

Dr. Ambedkar read the short file thoroughly. Ashoka then took control of the computer mouse and opened a window in which a series of 768 x 768 pixel CT images appeared, displayed using generic image software. Ashoka soon passed the mouse to Dr. Ambedkar, who scrolled through the images. He knew what he was looking for. The images followed one another rapidly, looking almost animated. In about ten minutes, Dr. Ambedkar went through over a thousand images stored in different folders. He also played twenty short films followed by a couple of X-ray images. Suddenly, Dr. Ambedkar signaled to Ashoka: he was ready to start the teleconsultation.

On the images reviewed by the pediatric cardiologist, one could see the heart of Mamadou, a nine-year-old boy who had been admitted a few weeks earlier at CHNU Fann. He was transferred from a hospital in Banjul, the Gambia. Upon arrival, Mamadou presented various symptoms including squatting, dyspnea during physical activity, and stunting. The antecedents of squatting and dyspnea went back several years. A clinical examination also revealed signs of cyanosis (bluish discoloration of the skin), deformation of the fingertips (clubbing), and the presence of a "precordial and left lateral sternal systolic murmur radiating to the back." Propranolol (a beta blocker) and a daily spoonful of iron syrup were prescribed to the patient. He also underwent a battery of tests: blood work, electrocardiography, an echocardiogram, an X-ray, and a chest CT scan. In light of the results, Fann's cardiologists diagnosed a tetralogy of Fallot with hypoplasia of the left pulmonary artery and partial anomaly of left pulmonary venous return.

Fann cardiologists were used to seeing and treating tetralogies of Fallot. Hypoplasia of the pulmonary artery, however, was much less common. For that reason, the treating doctor decided to present Mamadou's case during a staff meeting. The cardiologists present during the meeting suspected that they would have to transfer Mamadou's file to the Department of Thoracic and Cardiovascular Surgery. It seemed that a surgery would be inevitable. Even before the meeting, Dr. Leye, Mamadou's doctor, had discussed the case with a surgeon. However, neither the surgeon nor the cardiologists gathered knew how to proceed. First, they were not certain about the diagnosis. Then, the atypical nature of the condition could complicate any surgical intervention. They had never seen a similar case. A consensus emerged: why not ask "the Indians" their opinion?

As usual, it was Dr. Leye who went to the studios of the Pan-African e-Network to ask Jean-Louis if it would be possible to make an appointment with a pediatric cardiologist. He also wanted a pediatric cardiac surgeon to be present to discuss a potential surgical procedure.[11] Jean-Louis then sent a teleconsultation request to Ashoka by email. Technicians at the Fann and Apollo hospitals were used to working together. They preferred to communicate by email instead of using the chatting application included in the system. Jean-Louis would then input the patient's record to PAN's electronic medical records system. He attached the Word document prepared by Dr. Leye, to be read by Dr. Ambedkar. Jean-Louis also asked Dr. Leye to bring CT images and echocardiogram films using a flash drive. He later scanned the X-rays and transferred all the files via the network. At Apollo, Ashoka assembled all the documents. He inquired about the availability of Dr. Ambedkar and made sure of his presence at the scheduled time. Everything was in place for the teleconsultation.

After Dr. Ambedkar had finished looking at the images, Ashoka took control of the computer and opened the software (Polycom) used for teleconsultations. The teleconsultation was about to begin. Three people appeared on the screen. First, Jean-Louis and Dr. Leye. Then, a man introduced himself as the surgeon in charge of Mamadou's file. During the next fifteen minutes, he would not speak much or at least not directly with Dr. Ambedkar, preferring to ask Dr. Leye questions. After quick greetings, Dr. Leye and Dr. Ambedkar got into the thick of things. The Indian specialist confirmed the suspected diagnosis. He also insisted that surgical intervention was required as soon as possible. Dr. Leye inquired about the details of the procedure. Dr. Ambedkar gave precise directions on how to proceed. He explained everything carefully, making sure he was being properly understood. The discussion was open. Dr. Leye asked questions, made comments, and asked for clarifications. Dr. Ambedkar also asked questions, for instance about the patient's medical history. The discussion lasted about twenty minutes, after which the practitioners thanked each other. Ashoka then opened

VitalWare. Dr. Ambedkar took a few minutes to complete the "Opinion" section of Mamadou's electronic medical record, to leave traces of the teleconsultation. He wrote down his diagnostic impressions and the recommended treatment. Meanwhile, Dr. Ambedkar explained to me that he enjoyed participating in PAN. It felt like he was doing something useful. The network was working relatively well, he thought. There were not too many technical problems, and the schedule was convenient. Language was not a barrier either. His interlocutors seemed to have a good command of English. However, he noted, doctors from French-speaking countries often used French terms in the medical records, which was a little bit annoying.

A few months later, during my stay at CHNU Fann, I had the opportunity to review Mamadou's case with Dr. Leye. I wanted to know what had happened with the patient after the teleconsultation. Dr. Leye recalled that the Indian cardiologist had advised him to treat the cardiac malformation and then implant a stent in the branch of the hypoplastic pulmonary artery. After the teleconsultation, Dr. Leye and the surgeon on the care team consulted other colleagues to discuss the case some more. The surgeon discussed it with an anesthesiologist to see what risks of complications were involved in the intervention. They concluded that it was too perilous to have Mamadou undergo surgery at CHNU Fann. It was safer to transfer him to a better-equipped surgical ward. Because of the patient's young age, Dr. Leye explained, Fann's doctors thought that they could not do a complete repair of his tetralogy of Fallot. The presence of pulmonary hypoplasia changed the situation substantially since the surgical procedure would require a more complex intervention, with more hazardous resuscitation and surgery. The care team thus decided not to operate on Mamadou. The patient would be transferred abroad.

For many patients, Fann was a transit space. Mamadou had been transferred to Fann from a hospital in Banjul. After more than a month of undergoing medical examinations, his diagnosis was clarified and validated via PAN. Nevertheless, the DTCS team was not prepared to provide him with further medical care. As a result, Mamadou was only passing through Fann. When the care team decided against operating on Mamadou, they were under the impression that his medical insurance would cover his transfer to Europe. Transferring the patient to Dr. Ambedkar at Apollo Hospital in Chennai was not considered an option because insurance companies tend to have their own existing hospital networks for patient referral. In the end, it turned out that Mamadou's family did not have insurance to cover the transfer. The care team at Fann thus had to secure sponsorship to avoid sending Mamadou back to the Gambia without having received treatment. Ultimately, via the NGO Chain of Hope (the British version of La Chaîne de l'Espoir), Mamadou underwent surgery in the United Kingdom.[12]

The transfer of pediatric patients abroad was not rare at Fann. Mamadou's transfer indeed stood as a reminder of the institutional history of the Department of Thoracic and Cardiovascular Surgery. The DTCS started its activities in 2004, five years before PAN was launched. Until then, the Cardiology Department had seen pediatric cardiology cases, but its interventions were limited mostly to diagnoses. At Fann, in Senegal, and indeed in West Africa, this situation has been historically addressed in different ways. First, patients often received treatment abroad. Those with the financial means or those who are covered by medical insurance would seek care in Europe. Others were faced with very few options. In this context, NGOs have gradually developed humanitarian circuits aimed at providing medical treatment to young patients suffering from cardiovascular conditions. Since 1989, hundreds of children have been transferred from Senegal to Europe by charity organizations, the most prominent ones being La Chaîne de l'Espoir and Terre des Hommes. The case of Mamadou thus illustrates a typical North-South humanitarian logic by which the circulation of patients is the only way to get around local constraints and provide access to treatment.[13]

In addition to patient transfers, another key humanitarian response to the shortage of pediatric cardiology expertise has been overseas medical missions, with foreign medical specialists traveling to Fann to practice surgeries on patients. During my stay at CHNU Fann, for example, a surgical team from the Lausanne University Hospital (Centrie Hospitalier Universitaire Vaudois) in Switzerland was present. Composed of a pediatric cardiovascular surgeon, a cardiologist, an anesthesiologist, an intensive care specialist, an extracorporeal circulation specialist, and an intensive care nurse, the team came to operate on children with cardiac malformations. This was a humanitarian mission in good standing, organized jointly by the Lausanne University Hospital and the Fondation Terre des Hommes, an NGO specializing in child health. These visits are also part of what NGOs such as Terre des Hommes and La Chaîne de l'Espoir consider to be a change in approach, from the transfer of children to the transfer of skills. The approach, however, is not received with great optimism by all at Fann. Many doctors at Fann consider that these NGOs come with their own ideological agendas. As a cardiologist explained to me, they raise funds by turning the suffering of malnourished or dying children into a spectacle. Others suspect these funds to transfer patients to Europe are being "collected on the backs of Africans." Some even suggest that these patients are "good for business," given that they often suffer from pathologies with scientific value. Such skepticism vis-à-vis short medical missions is to be understood in light of broader postcolonial patterns of dependency and humanitarian circulation—after all, an organization such as Terre des Hommes has been involved in patient transfer in West Africa for over thirty years. Overall, despite the rhetoric of knowledge transfer and capacity-building, the humanitarian logic of the mission is slammed for its incapacity at building sustainable medical infrastructure, whether it be at Fann, in Senegal, or on the continent.[14]

To foster such long-term sustainability and decrease Fann's reliance on such humanitarian interventions—whether medical missions or patient transfers—the DTCS was created in 2004.[15] As a result, by the time PAN was launched in 2009, Fann was establishing itself as a regional hub for the management of pediatric cardiac conditions that required surgery. Pediatric surgery remained a poorly developed specialty in West Africa. CHNU Fann thus received patients from all over the region. But the DTCS remained a new department, and a case like Mamadou's came as a reminder of its persistent dependence on foreign aid and humanitarian circuits of care. But in spite of Mamadou ultimately being transferred to Europe, his case also testified to the relevance of PAN. What distinguished the services offered by PAN from other forms of circulation shaping the clinical space at CHNU Fann was a relationship between knowledge and space. Unlike the foreign doctor who occupied the clinic to operate on a patient or the patient who was moved out of the clinic, digital connectivity opened up the clinic and produced a space where expertise was always available and within reach. Instead of being sent away, complex patient cases became occasions to transfer knowledge and strengthen local clinical worlds. For Fann doctors, the transfer of *knowledge* ought to have been prioritized over that of *patients*. They considered the transnational circulation of knowledge a key strategy to empower local structures of care. In the words of Professor Bara Diop, "For us, it's a great project. They put us on the satellite. We are trained in a high-level technological environment. And the experience we capitalize on is an experience that we will use for our country. It's excellent for us."[16] Similarly, for Dr. Leye, the case of Mamadou was illustrative of the usefulness of the network: "You were there when we had this discussion, which brought us a lot of things. Because I knew nothing about the technique he mentioned. We can say, in medicine you do the courses and all, we teach you the cookbook. But not all recipes are in the cookbook! The great chef will always have a little recipe that belongs to him. Which is not in the cookbook! It's the same thing. There are cases sometimes, it is with the experience that one has it."[17]

The teleconsultation with PAN contributed to bringing about a new perspective on Mamadou's condition. While in a case like Omar's, the teleconsultation had reassured the care team of its ability to perform the procedure, the impossibility to care locally for Mamadou became obvious. In both cases, the effects of the network could be understood in terms of perspective or distance. At first glance, this seems to confirm a key expectation associated with PAN—namely, to facilitate the circulation of medical expertise by creating new South-South referral pathways. As mentioned in chapter one, PAN carried the promise that Indian and African hospitals were natural partners for medical cooperation due to an alleged resemblance between development trajectories. Ethnographic inquiry, however, complicates the naturalization of relationships between India and Africa. A case like Mamadou's, for instance, hints at the heterogeneity and indeed the overlapping—in PAN and beyond—of forms of travel between hospitals across continents. PAN got tangled with and ultimately fed into historical patterns of circulation—of knowledge and patients—that shaped medical care at CHNU Fann.[18] Even for those most optimistic about PAN, Mamadou's transfer to Europe served as a reminder of the persistent power of entrenched habits, pathways, and relationships.[19] But beyond this particular case, medical spaces in PAN were simultaneously bounded and permeable, composed of complex "alignments of materialities, social practices, and representations" (Street and Coleman 2012, 6). They were constituted by medical but also nonmedical material orderings of space. The next sections examine how PAN's clinic was shaped and held up from the outside—that is, from above and below.

Transnational Connections: From Above

The small bungalow lost in the Senegalese countryside looked pretty familiar. But despite its modest outlook, diplomats, ministers, journalists, and scientists frequently visited the site, where they would chat with managers and have their pictures taken. Located in Gandoul, about thirty miles from Dakar, the site was the cornerstone of the network infrastructure of the Pan-African e-Network. It was the Hub Center, also referred to as the Satellite Earth Station. The site that would become the hub of PAN's satellite network was selected following a call for tenders when the project was still on the drawing board. Many countries came forward with applications to host the hub and thus become the epicenter of PAN's operations. As it was explained to me by an officer at the African Union Commission who was involved in the process, Senegal was selected for three main reasons. First, Senegal was a coastal country with a landing point for submarine fiber optics—a feature that remained rare on the continent at the time that PAN was being designed (more on this later). Second, Senegal already had some experience with satellite technology, Gandoul itself having been home to a famous Satellite Earth Station since the early 1970s.[20] Finally, Senegal's principal telecommunications provider, Sonatel, already had plenty of experience with transnational networks, including managing segments between the landing station of undersea cables and satellite stations—a segment that was critical for PAN's infrastructure. Senegal, in my understanding, was selected primarily for historical and infrastructural reasons. These factors were considered more important than the fact that Senegal is a French-speaking country, which was a potential obstacle given that English was the working language of PAN. An official at the African Union Commission noted, "The English speakers didn't like it very much, but they won hands down, in a very open, well-done process."[21]

The Hub Center in Gandoul was built from scratch by TCIL in the months preceding the launch of PAN. By the time I first visited the center in 2011, it was humming with activities. Workers on the site included an engineer from Hindustan Computers Limited (HCL), the supplier of computer equipment for the project. The center had many servers, routers, and computers, which the engineer was in charge of maintaining. TCIL also had two employees on-site: an engineer responsible for the network and a supervisor coordinating the activities of the station. The primary responsibility of the Hub Center was to ensure that all of PAN's sites in Africa were properly connected. Tests between the TCIL data center in Delhi and the Hub Center were also carried out daily. The network was running twenty-four hours a day, seven days a week, regardless of its actual usage. Hence these three engineers lived at the station. They ate and slept there. Another engineer also visited regularly, working for the VSAT equipment supplier Nelco Ltd. (a subsidiary of Tata Indicom Telecom). Although he often traveled across the continent to oversee the implementation of the network, the director of African operations for TCIL was another frequent visitor. The Hub Center was divided into a few rooms. There was a main room with several computers, monitors, and satellite network resource management systems. The director had an office. Then there was the server room, bursting with servers, routers, and modems. All this equipment would have been of little use, however, if it had not been for the presence of a large Cassegrain parabolic antenna outside the station. The antenna pointed to the Rascom-QAF1R communications satellite in geostationary orbit. As the next pages suggest, the satellite is widely considered the central component of PAN's network infrastructure by the project's designers and implementers.[22]

Rascom-QAF1R was launched into orbit on August 4, 2010, by an Ariane 5 launch vehicle from the Guiana Space Center in French Guiana. Rascom-QAF1R was a replacement for Rascom-QAF1, the first satellite communications project dedicated to the African continent, launched in 2007. Rascom-QAF1 was operated and owned by the shareholders of the Regional African Satellite Communication Organisation (RASCOM), a pan-African organization of forty-five countries.[23] RASCOM was the first pan-African project to put a satellite into geostationary orbit and is often considered Africa's most ambitious postcolonial technological undertaking (Kane 2010). RASCOM's mission was first aimed at social and economic development.[24] Its satellites were to provide low-cost telecommunications infrastructure to facilitate the establishment of communications between countries and to offer a range of services to the population. Rascom-QAF1 was thus developed to support regional autonomy and cooperation. It sought to provide an African response to the Western domination of the satellite market. It would ensure a certain autonomy for intracontinental satellite links and thus avoid the use of the Intelsat satellite system, which is European and North American, to communicate among African countries (Fullsack 2012). In doing so, Rascom-QAF1 was expected to save annual costs of about US$500 million for the use of the Intelsat system.[25] It promised to connect remote areas and unify the continent through the satellite medium. So did its replacement, Rascom-QAF1R.

Rascom-QAF1's capacity to integrate the continent under its footprint was instrumental in making it a core element in PAN's design. PAN's designers at TCIL unanimously considered satellite connectivity the only practicable option to connect the African sites of the network. Also, Rascom-QAF1 was the only satellite available that covered the entire territory. These two criteria are worth examining in more detail. It should first be noted that satellite connectivity comes with significant drawbacks. Put simply, fiber-optic cables offer a faster connection, and with higher bandwidth, than satellites. They do not come with the kind of latency that is unavoidable with satellite technology. As we will see in chapter 5, latency has been a constant issue with PAN, especially for teleconsultations. The satellite thus slowed down the whole network, which could only be as fast as the slowest of its components. An engineer at the Hub Center explained, "The data is coming until Dakar in a IPLC [International Private Leased Circuit] network, and there is no delay. From there, from our Dakar station, it is boosted to the Rascom satellite. The delay is 200 ms. Then coming back to the remote station. Another 200 ms. There is no way around it. And it is working. You have to see the monetary angle, the coverage angle, and an acceptable delay. This is the best choice."[26]

Many PAN actors have emphasized the importance of the financial factor in designing the network. Although leasing satellite bandwidth can be very expensive, it remained much cheaper than laying a terrestrial fiber-optic network over the African continent would have been.[27] As was noted by Jean-Louis Fullsack, honorary deputy director of France Telecom, the need for satellite connectivity in Africa reflects the absence of a continent-wide fiber-optic network (Fullsack 2012, 102). For PAN designers, there was no existing terrestrial network infrastructure to work with, and laying cables across the continent was simply not financially or logistically reasonable: "The fiber was the best solution, but it doesn't exist everywhere. Satellite is easily deployable. Even within the country, within the city, within a few blocks, it would require an investment because sometimes you have a hospital site that is a little bit outside the city, the hospital not being connected to the fiber you would need to put that infrastructure in place. It would be very expensive. Whereas with an antenna, VSAT is easier to deploy."[28]

By contrast, satellite networks are much easier and cheaper to lay out. They only require installing Very Small Aperture Terminals (VSAT) at each point of service and monitoring the network from a Hub Center. Thus explained a TCIL officer: "VSAT is easy to install, and it is easy to establish the connectivity from any station to any station."[29] Small in size, VSATs were installed on the roof of hospitals participating in PAN. Compared to terrestrial lines, VSATs are portable and can be easily carried across geographical and political frontiers. Satellite connectivity, the TCIL scientist further explained, is advantageous in terms of stability as there is no risk of cable breakage or damage: "We don't have a single satellite connecting the whole world. That is the main issue. We have some satellites who will cover some parts of continents. We have chosen RASCOM, because it is the only satellite to cover the whole African continent."[30]

Rascom-QAF1 embodied PAN's ambition to rapidly scale the network, connecting over forty countries continuously. The project to unify an entire continent under the satellite's waves, which was made possible by its remote overhanging position, was inscribed in PAN's design. In contrast with the imagination of seamless global integration, however, PAN was the upshot of national and regional histories of infrastructure. This includes the history, recounted in chapter 1, of the development of satellite technology for telemedicine in India. In many ways, PAN would export—and showcase—the expertise acquired by the Indian Space Research Organization (ISRO) during the preceding decade or so.[31] A model for the private, vertical integration of health care, discussed in chapter 1, was also inscribed in the project's design. From the beginning, PAN would thus be a modern Indian experiment in Africa. PAN's infrastructure, however, was also rooted in regional African histories of connectivity. These include RASCOM's postcolonial development but also other more terrestrial genealogies of transcontinental connectivity.

. . . And from Below

When the time came to find a company to provide PAN's network connectivity within India, as well as between India and the African continent, TCIL—in conjunction with India's Ministry of External Affairs—issued another call for tenders. Bharti Airtel ultimately won the bid. The Indian telecom giant had vested interests in Africa. A few months after PAN's launch, for instance, it acquired

Zain Group's mobile operations in fifteen African countries, along with its forty-two million subscribers. The US$8.97 billion transaction, which had been years in the making, was India's second-biggest overseas acquisition ever. It gave a significant push to Bharti Airtel's attempts at breaking through into African markets (Banik and Nag 2016). It also made Bharti Airtel the world's fifth-largest wireless carrier by subscriber base and led to the foundation of Airtel Africa. Bharti Airtel's involvement in PAN thus did not come as a surprise, as it contributed to a broader movement of expansion and growth.

Bharti Airtel was responsible for connecting PAN hospitals in India using a fiber-optic network.[32] The hospitals were connected to a data center located within TCIL's headquarters in New Delhi. The data center comprised servers storing data related to the project,[33] a quality control room staffed by employees of i-Grandee Software Technologies (the company that designed the software used by PAN), and engineers who closely monitored the state of the Indian segment of the network. Bharti Airtel's role, however, was not limited to India. The service provider was also connecting India and Africa with fiber-optic undersea cables.

First, SEA-ME-WE 4 (fig. 3) was connecting India (Chennai and Mumbai) with Marseille, France. Spanning 18,800 km, the SEA-ME-WE 4 is a fiber-optic submarine communications cable system that carries telecommunications among thirteen countries over three continents. Laid in 2004 and 2005, SEA-ME-WE 4 is the primary internet backbone connecting Southeast Asia, the Indian subcontinent, the Middle East, and Europe. With an estimated cost of US$500 million, the contract for laying the cable system was awarded jointly to Alcatel Submarine Networks, France Telecom (now Orange), and Fujitsu Ltd. The consortium that is managing SEA-ME-WE 4 comprises sixteen international telecommunication companies including Bharti Airtel along with another Indian company, Tata Communications (previously government-owned Videsh Sanchar Nigam Limited, or VSNL). Bharti Airtel leased the bandwidth from SEA-ME-WE 4 for PAN. It also leased bandwidth from France Telecom for the European segment between Marseille and Lisbon, Portugal.

A second undersea cable system involved in PAN was ATLANTIS-2 (fig. 4), specifically its segment connecting Lisbon to Dakar. Commissioned in 2000, ATLANTIS-2 connects South America to Europe, passing through Cape Verde and Senegal. Costing over US$370 million, the construction of ATLANTIS-2 involved a consortium of some twenty-five service operators led technically and financially by Embratel, a major Brazilian telecommunications company (Sagna, Brun, and Huter 2013).

Importantly, when ATLANTIS-2 was inaugurated in 2000, Senegal was a forerunner in terms of transnational connectivity on the continent. ATLANTIS-2, in which Sonatel invested ten million euros, was the first optical fiber submarine

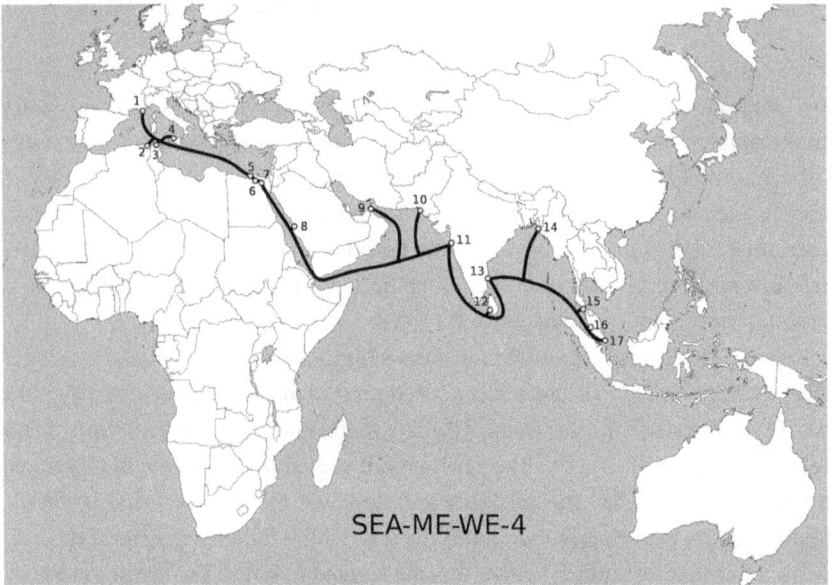

FIGURE 3. Map of the SEA-ME-WE 4 undersea cable route. Furfur (https://commons.wikimedia.org/wiki/File:SEA-ME-WE-4-Route.svg#file). Converted into black and white by the author. https://creativecommons.org/licenses/by-sa/4.0/legalcode.

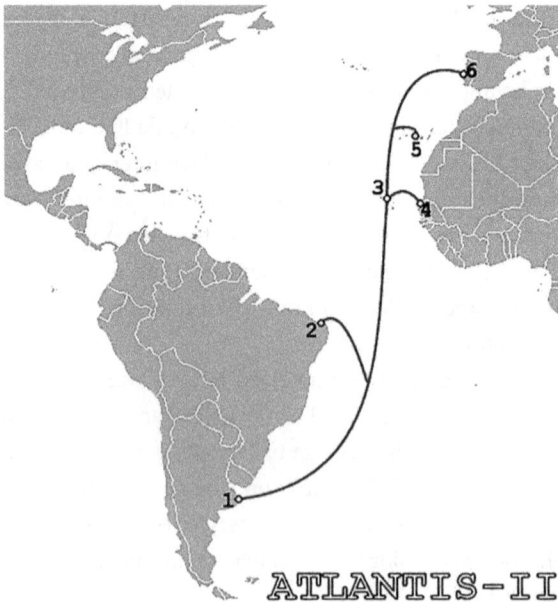

FIGURE 4. Map of the ATLANTIS-2 undersea cable route. J.P.Lon at the English-language Wikipedia. Converted to black and white by the author. https://creativecommons.org/licenses/by-sa/4.0/legalcode.

cable landing in Senegal at a time when few African countries benefited from such a digital connection with the world.[34] ATLANTIS-2 was a milestone in the development of national connectivity, the expansion of internet access, and a source of national pride in Senegal (Fall 2009).

As was noted by Lisa Starosielski, it is submarine systems and not satellites that carry most of the internet—more precisely, 99 percent of all transoceanic digital communications—across the oceans.[35] It is nevertheless important to keep in mind that when PAN was launched, sub-Saharan Africa remained relatively isolated in terms of undersea cable systems. It was served only by three submarine cables.[36] East Africa did not yet have any submarine cable landing, let alone a cable connecting with India. The rush to connect Africa had just started when PAN began its operations: between 2009 and 2012, several additional cables would be launched, with many more to come over the following decade.[37] Under these circumstances, bandwidth remained a luxury: bandwidth per capita in Africa was only 1 percent of the world average, and the continent had among the highest connectivity costs in the world (Juma and Moyer 2008). Not only were submarine cable landing points rare, but terrestrial national cable backbones were poorly developed. As a result, the continent remained the principal place where internet connectivity was primarily provided by satellite to avoid the high costs charged by network operators for access to international gateways to submarine cables (Malecki and Wei 2009).

The Pan-African e-Network thus embodied recent economic, infrastructural, and political histories of technological connectivity in Africa and beyond. Its design was contingent on the material conditions and the unequal topographies of global exchange by which some peoples and places were connected and others were not. However, the network infrastructure mobilized by PAN also came with unique promises of access, development, and economic growth. RASCOM emerged out of postcolonial, state-driven development politics, aiming to challenge Western-centric satellite markets. ATLANTIS-2 and SEA-ME-WE 4, by contrast, reflected the growing interest of telecommunication providers from the South, respectively from Brazil and India, in laying transoceanic cables and the related promises of integration into global circuits of capital and knowledge.

Network Labor and Care

At around 11:00 in the morning, the phone rang in the PAN studio at the CHNU Fann in Dakar. The call came from the Hub Center in Gandoul. The caller, a PAN supervisor, wanted to know whether it was possible for the TCIL engineers on duty at Fann to explain to a fellow engineer how to set up a teleconsultation. This was not the first time a supervisor had made such a request. The Hub Center was also the administrative center of PAN in Africa, and it would at times serve as an intermediary between hospitals. That morning, an engineer at the University Teaching Hospital in Lusaka, Zambia, had contacted a supervisor to ask for technical support: a doctor at the hospital, the largest in the country, wanted to use PAN for a teleconsultation in cardiology. The engineer in Lusaka, however, apparently did not know how to set up the teleconsultation. PAN engineers were supposed to receive some training from TCIL before being dispatched into the field. This had apparently not been the case for this engineer, who had just arrived in Lusaka. According to the engineers at Fann, situations like this were not rare. They did not mind it and considered it part of their job to help train newly hired colleagues.

A few moments later, the phone rang again. It was Vijay, the engineer in Lusaka who had requested assistance. Soon enough, Jean-Louis started giving him instructions: first, launch WinVNC, the remote computer control software. Jean-Louis and Vijay hung up and opened the software. They began to chat by typing short messages. From the beginning of the conversation, things were not going to be easy. Vijay manifestly knew little about PAN's computer platform. He did not know Polycom, the video conference software used for teleconsultations. He did not know how to select or contact an Indian hospital. Neither did he not know how VitalWare, the electronic medical record system, worked. Jean-Louis seemed a little discouraged. He knew the improvised training session would not be short. Below is a transcription of the beginning of their chat session (errors in the original have been maintained). The excerpts in lowercase were written by Jean-Louis, and those in uppercase were written by Vijay.

> ok sir wait a minute plz
> may i know your name sir ?
> SURE, MY SELF Vijay MAM
> OK HAVE U, U R NOT FROM SENEGAL HUB STATION?
> well i use to work there with them but actually i am in fann hospital
> where do u kept the data ?
> THE CD WITH DOCTOR ONLY. ACTUALLY U JUST INFORME ME
>   HOW TO DO
> sure i want to help but i need also to know what kind of data your doctor is having
> YES, SHE TOLD ME SHE SCANED THE PATIENT AND SHE HAVE
>   THE SCANED REPORT SO THEY THINK THE PATIENT NEED
>   OPERATION BUT BEFORE THE FINALISING THEY NEED
>   FURTHER CONSULTATION WITH INDIAN CARDIOLOGIST,
>   SO THEY CAME TO ME.

yes go ahead.

THIS IS THE FIRST TIME FROM ZAMBIA WE R DOING SUCH CONSULTATION, SO I WANT TO KNOW HOW WE DO CON- SULTATION, HOW WE UPLOAD PATIENT INFORMATION, IMAGE, SCANING VIDEO CLIPS, HOW WE GET ADVICE FROM INDIAN DOCTORS, HOW WE SELECT HOSPITAL,DOCTOR?

ok give me one moment

do u have polycom software ?

YES

WHY?WE NEED POLYCOME FOR CONSULTATION?

yes wOeK need it to interact with the indian doctor

but actually i need to talk with u,

look carefully what i am doing

HELLO?? MADAM???

i am not a madam

SIO RARM YA

R U GETTING ME ?

yes

SIR R U GETTING MY VIDEO AND AUDIO?

yes i am getting ur video and audio

do u have a camera by ur side?

YES

wait i will check the connection

give me 5 mins

OK

Jean-Louis and Vijay finally managed to speak together via Polycom. However, the quality of the transmission was not good. The image was blurred, and we could not hear Vijay, although he could hear Jean-Louis, who asked Vijay to adjust some parameters. After five minutes of unsuccessful attempts, the video remained erratic, but at least the audio was acceptable. The training session in due form could begin. First, VitalWare, PAN's electronic medical record system. VitalWare is a web-based application installed on a server in the hospital's server room. To access VitalWare, engineers had to first connect to the network. This required configuring the network's TCP/IP protocol on their desktop computer to include a valid IP address. Put simply, a device connecting to the network was not automatically assigned an IP address. The address, previously registered with the Hub Center's router, had to be manually input into the system. In theory, the computer could have been permanently connected to PAN to avoid configuring the connection every time. But the computer was also used to browse the web outside of PAN's network. PAN came with an internet connection. But some of the participating hospitals, like Fann, already had their internet access. And because the connection provided with PAN was particularly slow due to bandwidth limitations, engineers in hospitals like Fann preferred to keep using the hospital's connection instead. However, when the engineers wanted to use PAN itself, they had to connect through its satellite network to ensure the confidentiality of medical data. Hence the need to reenter the IP address into the system when connecting again.

Jean-Louis taught Vijay how to create a new patient record in VitalWare. He then instructed him on how to fill in the patient information and add text files and other relevant data. Often, doctors would send a Word document to the engineer: two or three pages summarizing the most important information in a patient's medical record. The engineer then simply attached this document to the electronic medical record. This is what Vijay did for that particular case, following Jean-Louis's guidance. Things were not so simple for images, however. Preparing for a teleconsultation usually involved the transfer of several images including CT, ultrasound, MRI, or X-ray images. Sometimes engineers would be given a compact disc or USB drive with the images. In other cases, they had to digitize the X-ray films that the physician had provided. Although this was not the case for Vijay, it was not uncommon that Fann engineers had to digitize images using the X-ray digitizer that came with PAN. The operation was both physical and software-based. Since there could be as many as twenty CT or MRI slices on a single film, after scanning, the engineer had to edit the images using software provided with the scanner. The engineer would cut the scanned film images into smaller images to reduce the size of the files before saving them. This was a tedious, time-consuming operation.

Ideally, patient image data would be handled in the DICOM format, which is the standard format for the management of medical images.[38] However, more often than not, PAN engineers had to work with images in the JPEG format. Differences between DICOM and JPEG are significant. First, unlike JPEG files, DICOM images contain metadata about the patient's case, such as clinical history or demographics. Second, the quality of the DICOM image is much higher. Certain aspects of DICOM images can be magnified by modifying the brightness or tinkering with the gray tones, thus offering more flexibility than JPEG files. The one significant advantage of JPEG is the file size. For example, a DICOM file including four MRI slices would be five or six megabytes (MB) in size—that is, several million bytes. The same image in JPEG format would be about two hundred to three hundred kilobytes in size, or a few hundred thousand bytes. According to Jean-Louis's experiments, a DICOM file would be over twenty-five times the size of the JPEG one. This is the only apparent reason why PAN engineers used the latter.

This technical choice introduces a major constraint of the network that engineers had to work with daily: limited bandwidth. Again, the teleconsultation that Jean-Louis helped Vijay set up was a case in point. The images that Vijay had to attach to the medical file were located on a CD that was provided by the physician requesting the teleconsultation. The CD contained several hundred images for a total size of nearly three hundred MB. Jean-Louis turned to me, looking doubtful: "This will never go through." He explained to his colleague, "You can upload up to fifty megabytes, but sometimes it will not work." The problem with uploading large files was that the transfer was too long, and the delay caused VitalWare to crash. In other words, Jean-Louis explained, attaching very large files to a patient's medical record was not possible. When the doctor arrived with either DICOM files or too many JPEG files, as was the case today, the engineer had to bypass VitalWare. The engineer then loaded the images into a folder on his workstation. He had to contact the colleague with whom he was setting up the teleconsultation in India to let him know where he had placed the folder in question. The colleague then downloaded the file to his computer using a file-sharing protocol. Bypassing VitalWare, however, could be risky: if a bug occurred on the computer, the images would be lost. Moreover, the transfer could still take several hours. However, there were few alternatives—bypassing VitalWare was often the only reliable way to transfer images that were essential for the teleconsultation.

Once the patient's medical file was completed, Jean-Louis further explained, Vijay had to make an appointment with a doctor in India. VitalWare was designed so that the teleconsultation request was part of the engineer's duties. After creating the patient's medical record, he would select a hospital from a drop-down menu with a list of every Indian hospital in PAN. Vijay told Jean-Louis that the doctor in his hospital wanted a teleconsultation with Apollo Hospital in Chennai. Once the hospital was selected, the engineer synchronized the record in the system. From a technical perspective, synchronization was the procedure by which the record became accessible to other hospitals in the network—in this case, Apollo Hospital. Synchronization could take some time. Often, the engineer had to make several attempts using files of varying sizes. It was some sort of a gamble: "Sometimes it will go, sometimes it won't."

Once the synchronization was over, it was time to contact the TCIL engineer at the hospital with whom a teleconsultation would take place. For hospitals with their own internet access, interactions of this type were typically done by email, outside the physical network of PAN itself. Vijay did not have the email addresses of TCIL engineers in India, so Jean-Louis gave him the email address for Ashoka (the engineer at Apollo in Chennai). He explained the steps to follow to finish preparing the teleconsultation. First, he had to contact Ashoka by email and inform him that he had just synchronized a medical record and requested a teleconsultation with Apollo. Ashoka would then log in to VitalWare and download the medical record. He would then make an appointment with a medical specialist within the hospital. At Apollo, this was done via the Apollo Telemedicine Networking Foundation (ATNF), which operates Apollo's nationwide telemedicine network within India and whose offices are next door to PAN. Medical specialists in India were generally very responsive and available on short notice. After hearing back about the availability of a doctor—in this case, a cardiologist—Ashoka would respond to Vijay by email. Several emails could be exchanged within a few hours. After the appointment was confirmed, Ashoka would prepare the patient's medical file and ideally share it with the doctor in advance. On another occasion, the doctors reviewed the file immediately before the teleconsultation, when entering PAN's studios. After the teleconsultation, Ashoka would open the patient's medical record in VitalWare so that the physician could fill out the "Comments" section with his or her opinion on the case discussed. Ashoka would then synchronize the file, update it on the network, and make it available to the treating doctors in Zambia.

PAN engineers were in charge of two main clusters of tasks. First, engineers had to maintain and operate the many pieces of equipment that came with the network. Every PAN site was equipped with video cameras, microphones, a projector, a digital production switcher, a printer, several servers, and routers. This was all professional, high-quality equipment.[39] To take the example of a hospital such as CHNU Fann, the computers were connected to the router located in the server room using standard RJ 45 connectors. Then the router was connected to a satellite modem that converted the satellite signal so that it could be read by the router. The modem itself was connected to the VSAT antenna installed on the roof of the building. Engineers made sure that everything was connected while remaining vigilant to detect any potential bugs. African hospitals were also provided with diagnostic equipment: a twelve-channel electrocardiograph, a mobile X-ray machine with a digitizer and darkroom equipment, an ultrasound machine, a polarizing microscope (for telepathology), and a glucose meter.[40] In theory, it was the engineers' responsibility to ensure that the medical equipment worked properly. But since they had not been properly trained to do so, it often proved challenging. When I asked the engineers at Fann how, if need be, they would operate the mobile X-ray machine themselves, they explained that it came with an instruction manual. PAN engineers had to learn rapidly and cultivate a sense of improvisation.

In addition to medical and computer equipment, all PAN sites, whether in India or Africa, were equipped with a set of three interconnected UPS systems to ensure that the network would operate for up to ten hours in the event of a power outage.[41] The system also protected the equipment from voltage fluctuations in the hospital's power grid. Although engineers monitored the network, they did not engage in any major repair work themselves. In the event of hardware failure or a computer bug, for example, engineers became intermediaries between TCIL on the one hand and equipment and service providers on the other. Engineers were tasked with monitoring and managing the network more than with actually repairing it.

A second set of tasks involved the daily administration of PAN's medical activities. Engineers played a key role in integrating the many components of the network: physicians, service providers, equipment, bandwidth, and the specificities of the connected hospitals (schedules, needs, etc.). Engineers planned and monitored the teleconsultations. They greeted visitors to the PAN studios. Engineers were TCIL's presence on the ground. They were the ones that physicians and hospital staff would go to with questions about PAN. In sum, engineers managed the day-to-day operations of the network, which could not be sustained without their labor.

This labor, however, was often monotonous, if not tedious. On both Indian and African sites, engineers passed time. It could be that nothing happened for long hours, especially when teleconsultations were scarce. At CHNU Fann, there were frequent visitors because the site was next to the hospital's other telemedicine activities. The atmosphere was good. In India, things tended to be calmer. Sometimes a doctor came in to give a CME session. At Apollo, there were also a few teleconsultations that filled Ashoka's days. Other Indian or African hospitals were seldom occupied. Overall, time passed slowly. Engineers got bored, especially those who worked alone on their site. They spent most of their days surfing the web, chatting, exchanging emails, or preparing for exams. They talked over the phone and listened to music. Yet the engineers I got to know were hardworking and ambitious. They considered their work on PAN a stepping stone to future careers and opportunities—more on this in chapter 4. If they were bored, it was because PAN ran at a slow pace. Their work was not only imperceptible, but it was also work of patience, routine, and repetition. It was far from the spectacle of a life-saving network; engineers were passing time.[42]

Fragile, Material Form

The clinic, argued Michel Foucault in *The Birth of the Clinic*, is to be understood as a site of validation for modern objects of knowledge and intervention (Foucault 1973). It is the site of the emergence of a medicine that is given and accepted as positive. The clinic, for Foucault, refers to a series of discursive practices that bring human lives within the reach of empirical knowledge. But medical knowledge, for Foucault, is always *spatialized*. Foucault has famously shown how the internalization of disease, and indeed of death, within the space of the individual body was instrumental in the birth of the clinic. It is only with positive medicine that "modern man" was offered "the obstinate, yet reassuring face of his finitude" (Foucault 1973, 193). In turn, this spatialization—in which the space of the body is enclosed in that of disease—is indissociable from a technology of the visible that he calls the "medical gaze." The medical gaze concerns the conditions of possibility of knowledge: it shapes the way we conceive, see, and speak about the human.

The persisting relevance of Foucault's analysis of clinical space lies in its attention to constitutive exteriority, making it impossible to reduce space-making to a process in which an "interior" (a clinical space, for instance) would simply emanate and grow *from within*.[43] The medical gaze does not refer to the act of seeing or to having access to something like a foundational subject of knowledge.[44] By contrast, because it always involves relations with outside forces, internalization is never a finite process. In Foucault's archaeology of medical discourse, there is no room left "for mystical interiorities, no tremulous interior self that was ontologically different from an 'object' exterior" (Farquhar 2016). Even in his early work on the clinic, Foucault challenged any notion of unmediated corporeal presence by which the clinic could be equated with a geographical space that would thus also obscure the tangle of human and nonhuman processes that generate and sustain life.

Digital technology in PAN transforms the conditions of possibility for medical knowledge and intervention—the modern clinic that Foucault described. This is true both of the conditions in which a diagnosis is made *and* of the therapeutic management of patient cases. As bodies are digitized and transmitted over the network, they are screened by a remote medical gaze with its own distribution of the visible and the invisible. The criteria upon which a body becomes the object of this remote gaze is no longer the expression of a localized illness but its communication over a great distance. Telemedicine produces a sphere of copresence in which the body's emergence as a site of intervention is freed from the imperatives of colocalization.[45] This emergence, however, is mediated by all kinds of technical processes. In PAN, nonclinical spaces, infrastructures, and labor are the source of medicine. The clinic, in PAN, is not a physical space in which technical operations would be carried out. Rather, the very possibility of medicine in PAN depends on the technical production of clinical space. This entails taking Foucault's cartography of the clinic one step further by opening it to the physical processes of networking, the enmeshment of things and peoples, matter and form. If we are to take seriously the ongoing process of formation by which the clinic comes into being, PAN can't be reduced to the assignment of an idealized vision or promise (the network form) upon materiality (the network, as raw infrastructure). Energy, practices of collecting, diagnosing, recording, transmitting, storing, and monitoring, need to find their way into the story.

Over the past few years, a wide body of work has attended to the mutual implications of the material and the discursive. Pioneering work in this regard includes early actor-network theory with its interest in the constitutive relations between humans and technology, approached as a material semiotics. As was described by John Law in a seminal article, material semiotics takes the semiotics insight, namely, that entities are produced and take their form in relation to other entities, "and applies this ruthlessly to all materials—and not simply to those that are linguistic" (Law 1999, 3). In dialogue with material semiotics, STS and anthropological studies of infrastructure have further challenged human-centric understandings of knowledge and care. Susan Leigh Star's work on infrastructure is particularly instructive in that regard. Infrastructure, for Star, refers to relational processes of sustaining worlds. It is relational in the sense that it "is something that emerges for people in practice, connected to activities and structures" (Star and Ruhleder 1996, 112). Infrastructure does not preexist the practices and things—patterns, habits, norms, material protocols, and tangible experiences and relations—that compose it. The same is true of a network infrastructure such as PAN. Star's work can be read as an invitation to think of networks in an ecological rather than a "connectionist" way that emphasizes only circulation and extension (Puig de la Bellacasa 2016, 53). As mentioned earlier, PAN was designed to be a scalable entity that would create new trajectories between India and Africa. This cutting of time and space into neat lines by the network, however, was contingent on the constant repetition of signals, labor, and technical routine.[46] Connections were built and sustained in practice through a careful, largely improvised work of articulation.[47] Once we pay attention to the background labor and processes through which a network like PAN is extended and stabilized, it becomes evident that the *structure* in *infrastructure* is solid only when seen from a distance (Berlant 2016, 394).

In recent years, "new materialist" work has further challenged human exceptionalism by insisting on the vitality of matter and things. New materialist writings have contested a dominant conception of matter as a fixed or inert substance. In keeping with such work, it is not possible to think about PAN in linear, productivist, or hylomorphic terms—namely, to start with a mental image and apply it to inert matter. The spatial ordering and discursive practices of the clinic were not fixed once and for all. Neither were they primarily human-based activities. They were, rather, following Karen Barad's proposition, "specific material (re)configurings of the world through which local determinations of boundaries, properties, and meanings are differentially enacted" (Barad 2003, 828). Stability and order itself were relational phenomena in PAN, drawing on specific maintenance and organizational activities (Denis 2019, 287). Despite—or perhaps because of—the dreams of grandeur inscribed in its design, PAN remained a fragile infrastructure kept afloat by repeated processes of trial and error. Very few things in PAN could ever be taken for granted. On a daily basis, thanks to the engineers' work, PAN was never completely broken. But as case studies discussed above show, PAN was also never completely functional. Things like technical glitches, disturbances, interruptions, and miscommunications were not external or opposed to but rather constitutive of network connectivity.

Inspired by new materialist writings, I thus do not approach PAN as a discrete entity that would connect preexisting material components, whether it be servers, wires, computers, or aerial and subterranean elements such as ATLANTIS-2 cables, terrestrial lines, and geostationary satellites. PAN is better understood as a material form entangled with messy and unsteady material ecologies, whose stability had to be enacted through continuous labor and care. Emphasizing the immanent relationality of matter, however, at times comes with a tendency to neglect material and discursive constraints and exclusions, whether they be historical, economic, political, topological, or otherwise. As the next chapter examines, PAN also came with affordances that generated transitory enclaves of care and shaped how peoples and places related to each other. Precarious material forms are also shaped by and can solidify existing power relations into consequential, even if temporary, spatial orderings.

3

THE ARCHIPELAGO OF CARE

A model is worked, and it does work.

—Donna Haraway (2016, 63)

When I arrived at the PAN offices at Apollo Hospital in Chennai, Ashoka was chatting with a Somali doctor who had requested an emergency consultation with a gastroenterologist. The PAN engineer in Somalia, Ashoka explained to me, was currently back home in India, on vacation. Since there was no one to replace him, he was now trying to guide the Somali doctor, Dr. Daar, in setting up the teleconsultation.[1] Dr. Daar readily followed the instructions provided by the engineer. While lamenting about the lack of a solution to replace absent engineers, Ashoka showed Dr. Daar how to log on to his account on VitalWare, the electronic medical record system. He walked him through the steps to fill in and upload the patient's health record. Once the record was completed, Ashoka told Dr. Daar to connect around 2:00 p.m., which would leave them half an hour to prepare for the teleconsultation scheduled at 2:30. Ashoka then called in an engineer working in the neighboring offices of the Apollo Telemedicine Networking Foundation (ATNF) who played the role of an intermediary between PAN and Apollo doctors. He wanted to make sure that the gastroenterologist contacted earlier in the morning would be present for the teleconsultation. The ATNF engineer reassured him: Dr. Mohan confirmed that he would be there on time, and he was trustworthy.

A little past 2:00 p.m., we connected with Dr. Daar. Ashoka explained to Dr. Daar that he wanted to check the quality of the sound and the video signal. As Ashoka completed setting up the teleconsultation, Dr. Jha entered the PAN premises at Apollo Hospital. Dr. Jha was scheduled to give a training session a little later, and he arrived in advance to prepare his presentation. Ashoka left the telemedicine studio to greet him and showed him to a computer in the adjacent control room. I stayed with Dr. Daar, who was waiting patiently for the beginning of the teleconsultation, with Dr. Mohan now running late. Dr. Daar explained to me that he was a newly graduated general practitioner and that he often used PAN to improve his knowledge and get support when he had questions about a patient. He usually asked for help reading electrocardiograms and ultrasound images. The network, he insisted, was a great resource. Dr. Daar practiced at Bosaso General Hospital, a public hospital in Bosaso, a town of seven hundred thousand in northern Somalia. Soon, however, our discussion was interrupted due to the poor quality of the signal. While the quality of the image and sound was very acceptable on our side of the network, Dr. Daar complained of a blurred image as well as sound distortion. Suddenly, an ATNF engineer walked in to let us know that Dr. Mohan would soon be with us. He had to perform an emergency surgery, and the delay was inevitable: "How can we say, 'Come to telemedicine?'" the engineer justified. Ashoka nonetheless regretted the delay. He explained that Dr. Daar had spent a lot of time preparing for the teleconsultation. The meeting, he insisted, had to take place as soon as possible since Dr. Daar's patient was currently hospitalized and had to travel several hundred kilometers to get to the hospital. Dr. Daar also considered the case to be a medical emergency.

Dr. Mohan arrived half an hour late at the PAN offices, apologizing for the inconvenience. The teleconsultation immediately began. Dr. Mohan started by looking at the images of the ultrasound before asking any questions of Dr. Daar. He preferred to verbally discuss the case rather than stick to the patient's medical record. Dr. Daar gave a lot of details about the condition of his patient. Many times, Dr. Mohan asked him what his clinical impressions were. For his part, Ashoka regularly returned to the studio to fine-tune the connection, especially the poor video signal. Dr. Mohan did not seem to mind the connection too much, even asking Ashoka to stop intervening: "Just let it go. Let it go." Having a conversation with Dr. Daar was more important to him than the quality of the image.

In her forties, the patient, Aasiya, presented symptoms of itching and severe abdominal pain. Dr. Daar also noted that her urine was brownish. Dr. Mohan suggested a diagnosis of dilated bile duct but insisted that it was impossible to detect the presence of stones or of a tumor in the images he was presented. The images lacked precision. Then the quality of the signal began to seriously deteriorate. Ashoka apologized and suggested that this was probably because Dr. Jha's CME session just started in the room next door, which used a lot of bandwidth. Gradually, the possibility of having a conversation became compromised: "Hello? Can you hear us, sir? Are you there, sir?" After a few minutes of trying to reestablish a good connection, Dr. Mohan was getting impatient: they still needed to discuss the diagnosis and the treatment plan. After one more relapse of the connection, Ashoka suggested opening a chat session so they could continue the teleconsultation in writing. Both physicians agreed. The session began with the gastroenterologist inquiring about the availability of certain drugs at Bosaso General Hospital. Here is a transcript of the discussion:[2]

> **APOLLO_CHENNAI-Dr.PC-03**
> ursodeoxy cholic caid
>
> **NEWUSER**
> no
>
> **APOLLO_CHENNAI-Dr.PC-03**
> antihistamines
>
> **NEWUSER**
> yes
>
> **APOLLO_CHENNAI-Dr.PC-03**
> use antihistamines
>
> **NEWUSER**
> ok
>
> **NEWUSER**
> how can i use the anti histamin
>
> **APOLLO_CHENNAI-Dr.PC-03**
> two times daily
>
> **NEWUSER**
> Avil 1x2 dialy [*sic*]
>
> **APOLLO_CHENNAI-Dr.PC-03**
> is there any possibility of CT Scan abdomen
>
> **APOLLO_CHENNAI-Dr.PC-03**
> ok u can use avil
>
> **NEWUSER**
> no in entire somalia there is no any ct or endoscopy
>
> **APOLLO_CHENNAI-Dr.PC-03**
> what is ur opinion on the USG

NEWUSER
dilated common bile duct

APOLLO_CHENNAI-Dr.PC-03
IF ANY OBSTRUCTION IN BILIARY SYSTEM U HAVE RELIEVE
    THE OBSTRUCTION BY SURGERY

NEWUSER
and u what is your openion in USG

APOLLO_CHENNAI-Dr.PC-03
otherwise the itching will not go

APOLLO_CHENNAI-Dr.PC-03
even i thought dilated bile duct

APOLLO_CHENNAI-Dr.PC-03
is there any possiblity of patient can come to chennai

NEWUSER
may be al will ask him [sic]

NEWUSER
do u charge him [sic] everything or for free

APOLLO_CHENNAI-Dr.PC-03
will charge only

NEWUSER
how can she come

NEWUSER
do u send the visa from ur hopsital

APOLLO_CHENNAI-Dr.PC-03
if she is willing we can arrange

NEWUSER
one minute i will ask her

APOLLO_CHENNAI-Dr.PC-03
ok

NEWUSER
3 questions

APOLLO_CHENNAI-Dr.PC-03
pl type it

NEWUSER
endoscopy how much, CT scan how much, and the visa how much

NEWUSER
i mean the charge

APOLLO_CHENNAI-Dr.PC-03
Endoscopie 30000, ct scan 15 000 visa i have to ask[3]

APOLLO_CHENNAI-Dr.PC-03
all these expenditure will send to you via email

NEWUSER
hello

NEWUSER
the patient says i can't come becasue of money

APOLLO_CHENNAI-Dr.PC-03
we will ask apollo Int.pat.dept to mail you

APOLLO_CHENNAI-Dr.PC-03
all amount quoted in RS.

APOLLO_CHENNAI-Dr.PC-03
in that case you go ahead with surgery

NEWUSER
ursodeoxy cholic caid, how can i use this, and what is this

NEWUSER
before the surgery

APOLLO_CHENNAI-Dr.PC-03
this is bile acid 300mg twice daily

NEWUSER
ok

NEWUSER
what is the benefit of bile acid

NEWUSER
in this case

APOLLO_CHENNAI-Dr.PC-03
it will reduce itching

NEWUSER
ok

NEWUSER
is this tab or what

APOLLO_CHENNAI-Dr.PC-03
ok thanks

APOLLO_CHENNAI-Dr.PC-03
tab

NEWUSER
send me all openions

APOLLO_CHENNAI-Dr.PC-03
ok

NEWUSER
thank you doctor

NEWUSER
for ur help

Chapter 2 explored how PAN made human life visible and accessible at a distance. I insisted on the materials and practices out of which network infrastructure emerged and clinical work was made possible. PAN, I suggested, was built out of relations, and its relative stability was enacted through continuous labor and care. In this chapter, I suggest that PAN did not merely connect remote locations but also produced distance between peoples and sites. The chapter examines the material form of the network. It explores how, in cases such as Aasiya's, mediation between medical worlds was hampered by the concreteness of place but also by the shape of the network. I suggest that the hub-and-spoke model of the network, which is at once a topological form and a market expansion logic, ordered the circulation of knowledge and constrained the possibilities for treatment. PAN, I propose, generated enclosures of expertise and care. Paying attention to the shape of the network and to its affordances prompts us to observe the relational, immanent power of materiality *along with* contractions, enclosures, and order-ings of various kinds. It raises important questions: What did the design of the network impose, and how it did it affect the making of global biomedicine in the context of South-South cooperation? How did PAN make certain things possible and not others?

Between Clinical Worlds

"It can become frustrating sometimes," Dr. Mohan disclosed to me after the tele-consultation. A frequent user of telemedicine, Dr. Mohan did not mind techni-cal issues. The medical constraints of the network, however, were tedious. Of particular concern were the clinical compromises that PAN kept forcing him to make. In almost every teleconsultation, he had to adapt to clinical settings very different from the conditions he normally worked in. He had to improvise, and this often led to diagnostic testing or treatment plans that he deemed inadequate. The case of Aasiya underlined some of the clinical constraints of PAN as well as potential adverse effects. First, there were material limitations. According to Dr. Mohan, the quality of the ultrasound images attached to Aasiya's medical file was not good enough. The problem was not one of resolution but of precision. The PAN engineer being on vacation, Dr. Daar himself had to operate the ultrasound system provided by TCIL, and he apparently struggled to do so. According to Dr. Mohan, he failed to bring out important elements: "I cannot see it," he explained. The gastroenterologist wanted to be able to rule out the possibility of a tumor. Then, as the chat session showed, it was not possible for Aasiya to undergo a CT scan of the abdomen without traveling. Clearly, Dr. Mohan did not appreci-ate practicing under such conditions. He explained that his Somalian colleague would have to operate on his patient without knowing what to expect. Was there an obstruction? What would he discover? The gastroenterologist insisted this was a relatively simple case for which making a diagnosis would take only a few hours at Apollo Hospital. Unfortunately, he lamented, medical expertise often can't overcome a lack of equipment: "They are still in the '50s or '60s in terms of medical facilities."[4]

The notion that Indian hospitals would be in a unique position to understand and adjust to the challenges faced by participating African hospitals was wide-spread among PAN actors including managers, politicians, and doctors. Accord-ing to a common narrative, the African hospitals connected to PAN were similar to what "Indian hospitals" used to be—that is, before the rise of corporate tertiary hospitals. In this developmentalist understanding of medical practice, Indian doctors were particularly qualified to take care of African patients by virtue of having, in the past, apparently practiced under conditions similar to those found in African hospitals in the present. Indian doctors, for example, would be experts in adapting to clinical environments with scarce resources and providing care to patients that couldn't afford the best treatment possible.[5] Indian doctors would have the appropriate experience and knowledge to adapt themselves and mediate between clinical worlds.

The reality on the ground, however, kept challenging this notion of a natural fit between Indian and African partners.[6] As is illustrated by the case of Aasiya, the conditions of everyday medical work in hospitals connected to PAN often shared little in common. It is also important to emphasize that Indian medical specialists participating in the project were most often seasoned physicians who had trained or practiced in the United Kingdom or the United States. Prior to PAN, they had practiced medicine only within corporate tertiary hospitals, with only a few having experienced public hospitals. While some claimed that being Indian helped them better understand the clinical reality of their African colleagues, the reality is that the material conditions of practice within a large Indian corporate hospital did not compare to those in most participating African hospitals.

In many instances, the very possibility of mediation between medical worlds was constrained by the materiality of place. Mediation was not restricted to the mere circulation of data and knowledge but also entailed dealing with wide disparities in terms of access to clinical and economic resources. Access to high-quality diagnostic devices (and the training to use them) or financial capacity to travel abroad and receive treatment were not evenly distributed over the network. As was explained by Dr. Faye from CHNU Fann, there is only so much that knowledge can do when detached from the material conditions of clinical practice:

> The problem is that sometimes it's not just the interpretation that is problematic. Sometimes it is the acquisition techniques and the performance of the device. It's because the device is not efficient. For example, there are 1 tesla, 1.5 teslas and all that. So, it gives you the power of the device. But to have the latest generation devices, you have to have money to do it! . . . We have devices that they used in Europe 10–15 years ago. So there are many things you cannot see. And we also have difficulties with the accessibility of these exams. There are certain diseases in neurology, if a patient for example has a stroke, it requires to make an IMR and a scanner upon arrival. In the minutes that follow. Here, it's downright impossible. So you are asked (by Indian colleagues) and then: 'No, it is not accessible!' In Senegal, there are three or four MRI machines. And for that, the patient is given an appointment within 2–3 weeks.[7]

Dr. Sow, also from CHNU Fann, concurs and emphasizes the discrepancies between the universality of medicine, understood as an abstract form of knowledge, and the concreteness of clinical work, which is to be situated in "the reality of the field."

> They can offer some form of explorations or treatments that are not available in Senegal. For example, immunoglobulin treatment is not available in Senegal! In our discussion, this is what they would propose to us. Like it or not, medicine is universal! Medicine, whether you go to Papua New Guinea, San Francisco or Dakar, in principle it should not be different! Now, these are the ways that differ! Someone may have cancer X, they need this type of chemotherapy. Whether in San Francisco, New Delhi or Dakar, theoretically it's the same thing. The Indian will offer us the same thing as the American, because it's universal! And we, if we had the same thing as San Francisco, we would have done this, but the problem is the reality of the field! It may not be available here. That there are substitutions they offer us is possible. If I cannot do it, I will see how to adapt to the current situation. There is nothing more human than that! This is the concrete part.[8]

Digital health often is associated with a promise to substitute flows of data and knowledge for the circulation of patients, the mobility of which is a common barrier to accessing quality health care. In PAN, however, it is clear enough that substitution is never total, nor is it generalizable. Medical expertise is produced on the network through constant mediation, by which knowledge is always transformed, and at times insufficient or inoperable. Sometimes, like in the case of Aasiya, data and knowledge travel across borders but capital, patient, and treatment do not. An excerpt from the chat between Dr. Daar and Dr. Mohan points to the crux of the problem: "The patient says I cannot come because of money." Discussing that situation, Dr. Mohan was straightforward: there should be ways to bring patients such as Aasiya to India and cover the expenses. Why, he insisted, invest so much in technology that enables patients to learn more about their medical conditions if we can't at least try to take proper care of them?

Aasiya's lack of access to treatment brought forth the situatedness of digital medicine, which entailed constant and constrained mediation between clinical worlds. Aasiya's case, however, was far from being unique. Many patients indeed learned about their medical conditions through PAN but without gaining access to treatment. PAN exposed and to some extent strengthened existing inequalities in access to care. This was not an anomaly but rather a feature inscribed in the design of the network. PAN made remote patients visible and accessible at a distance. It drew distant caregivers and institutions ever closer, bringing into intimate contact the suffering of remote strangers (Lock and Nguyen 2018, 292). The next sections examine how the intensification of global connections in PAN was structured by economic and network models, entangled in the design of the infrastructure. Specifically, PAN's capacity to do medicine was contingent on topological forms and a market expansion logic: a hub-and-spoke model that produced a series of spatial configurations best understood as connected enclaves of an archipelago of care.

A Hub-and-Spoke Model

"World-class, affordable healthcare is just 7 hours away," read the slogan on the Apollo Hospitals ad on the front page of the conference guide distributed to the visitors of the Ethio Health Exhibition in Addis Ababa. Designed to be a launch-pad for international companies looking to penetrate the market of Ethiopia and the East African region in general, the Ethio Health Exhibition is held once a year. In May 2011, the trade fair took place concurrently with the Second India–Africa Forum Summit, in Addis Ababa. The summit was the second in a series of offi-cial summits between India and Africa, the first one having taken place in New Delhi in 2008. The Ethio Health Exhibition is a large health care and medical international trade fair in which Indian hospitals play a leading role. The Indian government is a sponsor of the event. In the not-so-distant past, the presence of several Indian health care providers at a trade fair held in the Ethiopian capital under the theme "Health for All" might have come as a surprise. But when I attended the event in 2011, after spending a year on the traces of PAN, I expected nothing less from business representatives of Indian corporate hospitals. Pro-motional tours were indeed frequently conducted by Indian missions in Africa. Delegates from India had, for instance, visited CHNU Fann. Then, a few months later, health care was selected, just in front of information technology, as the top focus sector of the India Africa Business Partnership Summit held in Hyderabad in October 2011.

PAN was a public-private partnership funded by the Indian state to open new markets for Indian private hospitals in Africa. The project was launched in the context of the rapid globalization of the Indian corporate hospital sector over the previous decade or so. Around the time PAN was implemented, hospital chains such as Apollo Hospitals and Fortis Healthcare were rapidly becoming global play-ers in hospital markets.[9] Central to this global expansion was medical tourism—also referred to as *medical travel*—which describes the practice of patients traveling abroad to seek medical treatment.[10] Since the 1990s, many countries in the global

South had become valuable medical destinations, marking a shift "in international patient traffic from the global North to the global South" (Goldberg 2013, 1). Along with Thailand, Singapore, and Turkey, India soon became a leading worldwide destination for medical tourism (Chinai and Goswami 2007). In 2003, just a few months before PAN's announcement, Minister of Finance Jaswant Singh called for India to become a "global health destination" and pushed to facilitate the circulation of medical tourists, for instance by providing medical visas to foreigners seeking treatment in India.[11] By 2006, it was estimated that India welcomed about five hundred thousand foreign patients (MacReady 2007).[12]

The growth of medical tourism was supported by the Indian state, and corporate hospitals such as Apollo Hospitals, Fortis Healthcare, Max Healthcare, and Narayana Hrudayalaya rapidly emerged as industry leaders. Central to their growth was a capacity to provide treatment at a cost greatly lower than other competing destinations. For example, the cost of surgical intervention in India often was—and still is—one-tenth of the cost in the United States or the United Kingdom. Indian hospitals therefore like to advertise their capacity to offer what they often frame as "first-class treatment at Third World prices."[13] But as the slogan suggests, value is only one part of the equation. The Indian medical tourism industry also emphasizes the quality, carefulness, and safety of its services. Medical tourism advocates insist that the quality of medical care provided in tertiary Indian hospitals is comparable to the top institutions in the world. The quality of health care services, however, is not limited to medical expertise. Corporate hospitals welcome patients with marble floors, book cafés, a SIM card upon arrival, language interpreters, complimentary Wi-Fi, and overall superior accommodations. Medical tourism packages also often include spa treatments, yoga, or ayurveda as a way to entice tourists come to India. Most importantly, industry marketing insists on India as a place where caring is part of the national tradition, with a cultural predisposition toward providing care lovingly and compassionately. As was noted by Harris Solomon, both medical tourism advocates and foreign patients tend to "frame healthcare in the West as inconvenient, expensive, and often hopeless" while asserting "that India is a place to repair possibilities for hope and healing" (Solomon 2011, 106). This affective engagement with the nation as a "caregiver" is framed in terms that are at once patriotic and global, scientific and humanistic, commercial and benevolent.[14]

When PAN was launched in 2009, Western patients made up only a small percentage of India's international patients. Most came from neighboring countries, especially Bangladesh and Afghanistan (Connell 2006). But patients also were increasingly traveling from Africa to India to seek medical treatment. While the flow of patients from Africa was not a recent phenomenon, the number of Africans of non-Indian origins traveling to India for treatment started gaining pace in the early 2000s (Modi 2011). In East Africa alone, an estimated one hundred thousand patients traveled to India annually by 2015 to avoid long waiting lists and the high costs of treatment at home (The East African 2015). In 2015, East Africans spent around US$1 billion on Indian health care (Mitchell 2017). Driven by global disparities in access to tertiary care, the rapid growth of "South-South medical tourism" (Ormond and Kaspar 2018) has drawn criticism for encouraging the outsourcing of medical expertise rather than the development of local capacity.[15] For African patients, doctors, and hospitals, medical tourism produces a new form of dependency on foreign expertise and institutions. For corporate hospitals, on the other hand, it is a key component of market expansion and the creation of a transnational pool of middle- and upper-class patients wealthy enough to afford treatment.

By the time PAN was launched, however, the expansion of Indian corporate hospitals in Africa was not limited to medical tourism. In addition to treating patients coming from all over the world, Indian hospitals had started engaging in a whole array of commercial activities in Africa. Chains such as Apollo and Fortis opened new hospitals, set up joint ventures with local health care providers, offered consultancy services, and trained doctors, paramedics, and national health ministries.[16] Corporate hospitals aimed to export to Africa a business model developed within India and revolving around a strong referral network whereby smaller institutions in semiurban, rural, or remote locations would screen patients and refer them to "hub" hospitals in Indian metropolises. Commenting on Apollo's expansion in Africa in particular, Preetha Reddy, managing director of Apollo Hospitals, referred to this as a "hub-and-spoke model" in which the centers with lesser facilities are supported by comprehensive tertiary care hospitals—of which Apollo hospital in Chennai stands as a flagship illustration (Babu 2014).[17]

The hub-and-spoke model promoted by Preetha Reddy is a well-known model for the distribution of health services and market expansion. As I will explain later in this chapter, hub-and-spoke is simultaneously a business model and a network topology by which PAN organized the spatial relations between its nodes. The hub-and-spoke model was key to the development of telemedicine in India in the years preceding PAN. As discussed in chapter 1, telemedicine played a key role in setting up referral networks between health institutions and providers across India. For patients, telemedicine lowers the costs that come from seeking treatment, including transportation expenses, and lost wages during time away from home. But it also establishes contact between doctors, creates referral patterns and routes, and ultimately builds a patient pool by connecting remote doctors, patients, and institutions. As was suggested in a paper published in the *Harvard Business Review*, telemedicine, along with the hub-and-spoke architecture developed by Indian hospitals, helps create large volumes, allowing hospitals to reap economies of scale and to make the business profitable (Govindarajan and Ramamurti 2013).[18] The same model applies to the expansion abroad of Indian corporate hospitals. Dr. S. K. Mishra, a pioneer of telemedicine in India, explained to me how deeply entangled telemedicine and medical tourism are: "Telemedicine has helped in facilitating this going overseas. Medical tourism has a lot to do with telemedicine. . . . First, there is pre-referral screening. 'I talk to you, I tell you a problem, my images are seen by you.' So I should get their scans and everything before they are coming here. By connecting to this doctor, I get customer satisfaction. I just reached at this stranger and if you need a surgery, you want to go see that doctor. This is pre-referral screening. This is what I do day in and day out here."[19]

Telemedicine builds trust in relations to come. It facilitates market expansion, to which Apollo Hospitals' chairman Prathap Reddy earlier referred to using the notion of "vertical integration." As the case of Aasiya showed, not every patient in need of medical treatment could travel via PAN. Other patients like Mamadou, discussed in chapter 2, traveled abroad for treatment following a teleconsultation with PAN but not to India. The recourse to older humanitarian routes made visible preexisting patterns of circulation at CHNU Fann and beyond. However, in many other cases, PAN *did* encourage patients to seek treatment in India and fostered medical tourism. The exact number of African patients who traveled to India via PAN is hard to verify. An engineer who was posted in several countries to work on PAN retrospectively mentioned having witnessed or helped facilitate hundreds of patients traveling. Others had not heard of any. TCIL officials would speak of medical tourism as an important spin-off of PAN, also citing hundreds of travels. Speaking about the hospital's participation in the project, a manager at Narayana Hrudayalaya in Bangalore suggested that PAN fostered expansion and growth: "The project is saying that India has got 12 hospitals for the whole of Africa, who can take care of expert opinions, who can take care of surgeries which cannot be performed in Africa. You can come here and get your surgeries done and go back. It is all about it. That's how I would define 'growth.'"[20]

In PAN, the hub-and-spoke model was central to the imagination of growth and expansion. The adoption of this model enabled the connection of distant hospitals, thus reaching patients rich enough to travel to India while bypassing other "irrelevant" people and places. The economic potential of PAN lay in its capacity to integrate remote places into a transnational space of circulation for beings and things. To borrow from the anthropologist James Ferguson, the movement of capital in PAN was globe-hopping, not globe-covering (Ferguson 2006, 38).[21] Similarly, anthropologists of global health have challenged a prevailing imagination of transnational mobilities and connectivities in terms of flows.[22]

Anthropologist Wenzel Geissler, for example, has suggested that science and public health in Africa take the form of an archipelago of connected yet insulated sites through which expertise, data, and resources circulate without "touching upon national structures of knowledge generation and use" (Geissler 2015, 14). Writing about the changing landscapes of medical research and public health in Africa, Geissler invites us to consider how new economic forms in global capitalism are accompanied by spatial change, including in health care. We have moved away, Geissler notes, from past imaginations of social, political, and economic action as an expansive movement from the center outward in which space was being appropriated through back and forth between center and periphery, and distant places were integrated into a "concentric functional whole" (Geissler 2014, 231). Reflecting these broader changes in global capitalism, public health science in Africa is no longer characterized by stable spatial and political form—for instance, by the nation-state—but rather by fragmentation and insulation: by "enclosures, exclusions, hopping connections, and ephemerality" (235). However, Geissler insists, relations in this new fragmented geography remain asymmetrical: "Inside and outside are not equivalent positions toward enclosures; and connections are initiated, controlled, and sustained from certain locations and positions of interest and ownership" (232). In the following sections, I examine the entanglement of connection and insulation in PAN and how it enacted asymmetrical relations. I suggest that building global connections depended on fencing off PAN from the many environments in which it was installed at organizational, spatial, and topological levels. It entailed spacing. This distance was not accidental, I suggest, as it was purposefully inscribed into the design of PAN.

The Shape of the Network

In the heart of Addis Ababa, the Black Lion Hospital is the largest public hospital in Ethiopia and one of only two university hospitals in the country. Built on seven floors, and with over eight hundred beds, the hospital is immense. When I first came to the Black Lion, I soon realized that finding the PAN installations was no small feat. Employees at the hospital's reception desk were not aware of the studio's existence. After wandering around the hospital for some time, asking for directions, I finally found the PAN studios at the end of a poorly lit, deserted corridor on the second underground floor of the hospital. Entering the installations was like entering a different world altogether. The quietness of the room stood in contrast to the effervescence observed in the other departments of the hospital. The contrast between an abandoned corridor with cables hanging from the ceiling and an air-conditioned room equipped with state-of-the-art computer equipment was also striking. Although the room was smaller than the one at CHNU Fann, there were still about fifteen chairs in the room for attendees of the CME sessions. The telemedicine studio had been set up in an adjacent room. One engineer spent his days there, with plenty of time to make sure everything was in order.

The Black Lion Hospital was not an exception: In every hospital I visited, PAN installations were spatially isolated from the surrounding hospital activities. PAN operated in physically remote sites located on the periphery, insulated from the hospital wards and their everyday operations. This also was the case in India. For example, at HCG Hospital in Bangalore, the project occupied a newly built space on the roof of the hospital. Most of the time, PAN was located adjacent to the hospital's national telemedicine program. Yet regular telemedicine activities are usually cut off from the rest of the hospital in some way. They are not integrated into a particular department; they occupy premises that are entirely dedicated to them. Hospitals generally chose to expand or vacate facilities to accommodate PAN by adding another room exclusively for TCIL use. As a result, in terms of spatial organization, PAN was partly if not completely isolated from the rest of the hospital. It was not a site through which one ordinarily went without a purpose. Like at Black Lion, many did not even seem aware of the existence of the site. PAN, I suggest, actively insulated itself from the environments in which it was operated. The distance was physical but also logistical and organizational. As mentioned earlier in the book, PAN came with a "portability kit" that included UPS systems, on-site installation standards (e.g., air conditioning, plenty of work-spaces, etc.), medical and computer equipment, and a mobile workforce (e.g., engineers and managers). The kit itself was part of a wider turnkey approach by which labor force, materials, and protocols would be delivered by TCIL as part of a standardized package.

However, spatial isolation and organizational standardization are not suffi-cient to understand how PAN managed relations between people and between people and things. It is important that we also pay attention to the shape of the network and specifically to the hub-and-spoke topology, also known as a *star topology*. Steven Connor, in a commentary on the work of French philosopher Michel Serres, suggests topology is the study of the spatial properties of an object that remain invariant under actions of stretching, squeezing, or folding. Topology is concerned with "spatial relations, such as continuity, neighbourhood, inside-ness and outsideness, disjunction and connection" (Connor 2002). Network topology in particular is best understood as the topological structure of a com-puter network. It is a physical and logical arrangement of nodes and connections.

In examining PAN's network topology, particular attention shall be given to satellite technology. As explained in chapter 2, to connect participating hospitals,

PAN relied on the Rascom-QAF1R satellite, whose footprint covers the whole African continent. However, the possibility of satellite unification of the continent came with a serious topological paradox. On the one hand, by physically connecting very distant sites, the satellite fueled the imagination of a unified space. Distant colleagues and patients appeared to be effortlessly available, and connected sites were turned into manageable nodes in a networked world. The satellite seemed to be the ideal medium for the "vertical integration" dreamed about by Dr. Reddy, among other telemedicine enthusiasts. On the other hand, remote communication in PAN depended on a centralized controlled network infrastructure materialized in its topological form. The design of the network form deserves some attention.

Satellite networks are most often designed according to one of two types of topologies: hub-and-spoke and mesh topology. In a hub-and-spoke topology, all communications pass through a hub that acts as the network's control center, connecting the nodes—specifically, the VSATs—through the satellite. Conversely, in a mesh topology (also called *point-to-point*), each node is directly connected to another node through the satellite without going through the hub. There is no central point, no hub, and all the nodes are connected in a meshlike structure. These two topologies come with their advantages and drawbacks. First of all, a mesh topology undoubtedly offers better performance in terms of connectivity. The connections between the nodes are more direct and faster. In contrast, with a hub-and-spoke topology, each communication between two nodes is subject to a double hop since each node must pass through the hub before communicating with the other. As a result, both the latency time and bandwidth usage are doubled. Hub-and-spoke topologies are therefore generally not recommended for video applications such as medical teleconsultations (Graziplene 2009). Furthermore, in a hub-and-spoke topology, the total bandwidth of the network is limited by the capacity of the hub. As the number of devices connected to the hub increases, the total bandwidth of the network may become limited by the capacity of the hub. This can lead to congestion and slow network performance.

A mesh topology also provides greater stability since it does not depend on the proper functioning of a hub that can quickly become the nerve center of the network. In the case of a hub-and-spoke topology, if the hub fails, then the whole network fails. In contrast, in a mesh topology, each node has its own hub, so to speak: a service outage won't affect the entire network. While this relative autonomy of the nodes is an interesting advantage of the mesh network, it is also accompanied by an important disadvantage: cost. Indeed, in a mesh topology, each of the nodes must be equipped with a significantly larger antenna as well as an expensive satellite modem. For a satellite network, a mesh topology can therefore require a huge upfront investment. In a hub-and-spoke topology, in

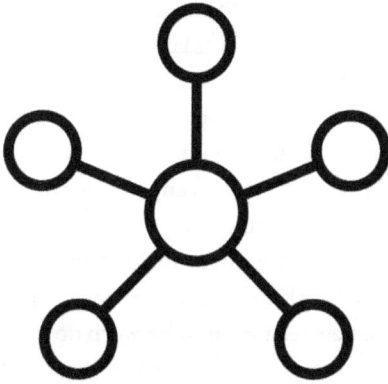

FIGURE 5.   Diagram of a star topology.

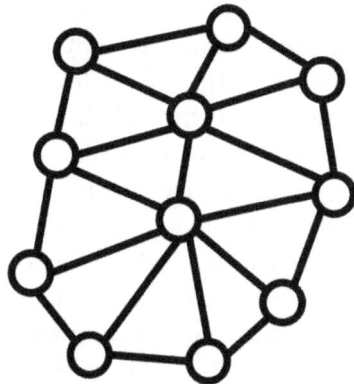

FIGURE 6.   Diagram of a mesh topology.

contrast, the hub is equipped with a high-powered antenna (nine meters) while the VSAT antennas used on every site (i.e., the hospitals) are much smaller, varying between one and three meters (2.4 m in the case of PAN). By choosing a hub-and-spoke topology, PAN designers were therefore making a sound financial decision.

Perhaps the most important quality of the hub-and-spoke topology as far as PAN was concerned was centralized control. Because all devices were connected to a single hub, it allowed for easy management and control of the network. This helped prevent any unsolicited connection to the network: the hub ensured control of all transmissions (Elbert 2004, 297). For this reason, while the mesh topology is generally recommended for bandwidth-intensive point-to-point interaction (such as video), the hub-and-spoke topology is often recommended for networks where sensitive data circulate (e.g., corporate networks). Because of the centralized spatial distribution afforded by a hub-and-spoke topology, TCIL could ensure a high level of control over the medical data flowing via the PAN network. The hub-and-spoke topology is particularly amenable to some form of centralized control and governance.[23] In PAN, this was often referred to in terms of security.[24] Put roughly, the hub-and-spoke topology enabled the Hub Center, in Gandoul, to control the circulation of data, manage its encoding, and assure its security. It was an obligatory passage point. As it translated between satellite and optical fiber, the signal was encrypted. In the words of a TCIL executive, the Hub Center acted as "an Indian gateway into Africa."[25] As a result, PAN was at once extensive and centralized; it was wireless but accessible only from specific sites with the help of precise equipment and on the condition of being in possession of certain codes and privileges (frequencies, passwords, etc.). While the network enabled a virtual opening of the clinic, the opening was possible only on the condition of a whole series of affordances and exclusions. Through topological form and security processes, PAN's network boundaries were actively managed and guarded against any potential outside activities or interference. For example, participating hospitals were prevented from exchanging data or expertise directly with each other without going through the hub, thus foreclosing potential unplanned collaborations. Connectivity in PAN was engineered so that certain relations were enabled or valued while others were not.[26]

In PAN, the promise of market expansion was contingent on making new bodies visible to knowledge and intervention. Network infrastructure would open hospitals to a world of expertise and cultivate new relationships between doctors, some of which would lead patients to travel abroad. As discussed in chapter 2, this opening of the clinic was contingent on materialities but also on the constant work of mediation by which boundaries were drawn and interior spaces were generated. However, the ordering of movement and the production of space in PAN were to a large extent inscribed in the shape of the network from the design stage. This is where network topology comes into play. Put simply, the hub-and-spoke topology materialized, in network form, the business model promoted by Apollo Hospitals. It was imagined as a privileged medium to build a larger patient pool through the circulation of expertise and technology.[27] Network form and economic model were deeply entangled in the design of PAN as hierarchical and differential network structures aimed at geographic expansion.

Direction and Authority

Dr. Roy was excited when he walked into the studios of the Pan-African e-Network at around 3:00 p.m. The neurosurgeon had been conducting teleconsultations for years. However, it was easy to sense that he was feverish about one in particular. A few hours earlier, Ashoka, the PAN engineer on-site, had asked to see him. He wanted to get Dr. Roy's opinion on a teleconsultation request that was waiting for him when he arrived at work in the morning.[28] When Dr. Roy came in, Ashoka presented him with a series of CT images of a brain. The neurosurgeon quickly scrolled down the images on the screen, all in JPEG format. He then stopped short and told us that he had never seen an intracerebral hemorrhage of this type, presenting such a pattern. He replayed the images on the screen and finally asked Ashoka to transfer some of the images to him by email. He wanted to ask a radiologist friend his opinion. He insisted that the engineer should send him the images right away, to give the radiologist enough time to review them before the teleconsultation, which would most likely take place on the same day. It was almost noon when Ashoka transferred the images to Dr. Roy, who had left the PAN studio as quickly as he had arrived.

Dr. Roy came back to the studio at around 3:00 p.m. He was accompanied by a visitor from the Apollo TeleHealth Services (headquartered in Hyderabad), Apollo's commercial telemedicine wing. Dr. Roy wanted to show his guest some of the telemedicine work carried on at Apollo Hospital, including the Pan-African e-Network. The neurosurgeon was particularly agitated, primarily because of the apparent rarity of the case under study. Dr. Roy is passionate but also voluble, with a keen sense of performance. When he entered the PAN studio, Ashoka was already in conversation with Jean-Louis at CHNU Fann. The quality of the video was particularly good. The sound, however, was poor. The latency in the transmission was awkward, and there was distortion. To partially mitigate the situation, Ashoka used a headset. In the back, at CHNU Fann, Dr. Faye and a colleague were already present and waiting. Dr. Roy then entered the telemedicine studio. The neurosurgeon took a seat behind the monitor, and the teleconsultation began right away.

The greetings were brief because a radiologist arrived at the same time in the PAN studio. Dr. Bose was coming in a little early to prepare a CME session she was about to give on the topic of "Interpretation of Spinal X-Ray." Visibly excited by this impromptu arrival, Dr. Roy invited her to join the teleconsultation: he would love to have her opinion on the case being discussed. Dr. Roy asked Ashoka to put the CT images back on the screen. Ashoka apologized quickly to our Senegalese interlocutors before doing as told. Then, for several minutes, Dr. Roy and Dr. Bose discussed the images. Dr. Roy suggested a diagnosis. He regularly turned to his guest and myself to comment. He explained that this was a case that was rarely seen in India, but he believed it was more common in Africa. Dr. Bose seemed hesitant about the diagnosis and suggested other options. Suddenly, someone pointed out to Dr. Roy that the microphone was left on and that our Senegalese interlocutors had thus been listening to the whole discussion. The neurosurgeon did not make a big case out of it: "They do not understand us anyway," he explained, confident that the Senegalese doctors on the other side of the screen did not properly understand English. Dr. Bose then left the studio to go prepare her PowerPoint presentation in the room next door.

After Dr. Bose left, Dr. Roy, confident about the accuracy of his diagnosis—which he had come up with while discussing it with another radiologist earlier in the afternoon—finally addressed the CHNU Fann team, still waiting on the other side of the screen. The neurosurgeon spoke loud and fast. He presented his diagnostic impressions with confidence and authority. Because he was wearing headphones, it was difficult to hear what his interlocutors were saying, but they did not get the chance to intervene much. After a few minutes of a teleconsultation with the appearance of a soliloquy, Jean-Louis asked to speak with Ashoka. The latter then seized the headphones. Moments later, he removed them and spoke to Dr. Roy: "Sir, they want to know if you can speak slower." Dr. Roy then put the headphones back on and started talking again, only much slower. He made an effort to be better understood. Nevertheless, based on the body language of the Fann team, it was obvious they were still having a hard time understanding what Dr. Roy was saying. After they signified their incomprehension, he instead began to write his clinical observations in the patient's file, in VitalWare. Dr. Roy removed the headphones and focused on this task. When I asked whether the Fann team would be capable of understanding his written report and whether he'd like me to help translate some key terms in French, he declined the offer and reassured me, "Do not worry. They understand. I just wrote the report."

Before closing the teleconsultation, Dr. Roy put the headphones back on. With great enthusiasm, he started talking again at an accelerated pace. He entered the heart of what, for a few hours, had aroused his enthusiasm. The neurosurgeon began to explain to his colleagues at CHNU Fann how rare such cases were in India. They should, he insisted, publish a scientific article based on the case: "You could be the first author. This is a rare case. An international case." He then asked the treating doctor at Fann to send him the results of the patient's biopsy so they could move in that direction. He insisted that we take pictures of him in front of the screen, explaining that this would now be a case he could use in scientific conferences. According to Dr. Roy, this case was a success story that deserved publicity: "When you go back to Canada, you can tell them that we are really doing something in this project. Things are really happening." Certainly, the neurosurgeon was taking pride in having possibly solved an "international case." He then rapidly left PAN's studio, visibly satisfied.

The scene described above brings out different elements that I have encountered frequently in observations and interviews in a particularly vivid way. First, there is the asymmetry of the exchanges. During the teleconsultation with Dr. Roy, the communication was unidirectional: the neurosurgeon was giving his opinion. When I pointed this out to Ashoka, he suggested that Dr. Roy could behave this way because of his experience and seniority. Doctors and engineers at Fann later agreed that the specialist's attitude could be explained by a "generational issue." They considered, however, that this was not ideal. Dr. Roy always seemed to be in a rush, and he reprimanded them whenever there was the slightest delay in the schedule: "We feel like he's always in a hurry. Well, that bothers us because he comes quickly, he does it quickly, he leaves, he yells, he screams. Frankly, it's difficult with him."[29]

This performance of authority by Dr. Roy challenged ideals of horizontality and mutual exchange that are key to the promise of South-South cooperation. Mutual exchange, doctors at CHNU Fann insisted, is a bulwark against the instauration of dependence on outside expertise. To avoid this trap, Fann doctors prepared their cases well: they discussed among themselves, looked up the literature, and got ready to potentially challenge the opinions received via PAN. Fann doctors approached knowledge production as a shared, distributed process. Here is Dr. Diop: "These are exchanges. And we often come (to PAN) because we have an interesting case, we know what it is, we know how it can be treated, and we come. . . . We teach them, there are things that we teach them. You'll ask Dr. Roy, he'll tell you that there are cases that we've presented here that they've never seen before and that they're learning something. That is to say that officially there is this paternalistic approach, but in fact there are many things that we also bring to them in terms of experiences."[30]

Dr. Diop thus insisted on the reciprocity of exchanges. He was confident that from the seemingly disembodied ritual of teleconsultation, some kind of scientific complicity, if not an epistemic community, could emerge.[31] This is what Dr. Roy seemed to suggest when he mentioned the joint publication of a scientific article based on the case discussed during the teleconsultation. However, Dr. Roy's performance in the telemedicine studio *also* suggested a much more unidirectional and indeed authoritative approach to the making and exchange of expertise. This is partly due to Dr. Roy's personality but also to hierarchies that are ubiquitous within hospital environments. It also, I suggest, illustrates asymmetries that are underlying teleconsultations in PAN. As reported by another physician at CHNU Fann, "Very often what happens is, you write your case, you send it, they read the case and then the day you come, they tell you what they think. So it's not so much a dialogue! They ask you questions, 'Is there this, is there that?' And then you say, 'No, no, no.' Then they tell you what they think and that's it."[32]

Under these conditions, the spirit of transnational collegiality among colleagues developed slowly, if at all. With few exceptions, relationships among physicians did not extend beyond the framework of teleconsultations. The vast majority of physicians did not seem to know the names of the colleagues with whom they were doing teleconsultations. They often knew very little about the hospitals they were in contact with. For example, they might have thought that Apollo Hospital was in Mumbai or that AIIMS was a private institution. Similarly, Indian doctors often could not differentiate between the hospitals connected to the network or even the countries where they were located. Overall, most of the teleconsultations taking place on PAN were to a large extent anonymous. This anonymity was not neutral. In many ways, it was a display of authority. Moreover, the teleconsultation with Dr. Roy pointed to another manifestation of anonymity: the nameless patient. Despite the rarity of his condition in the eyes of Dr. Roy, he never asked for any information about the patient. Dr. Roy knew he was a ten-year-old boy, and that was it.

What is interesting here, however, is not so much what is lost in this process of objectification—the patient reduced to his or her body, to the images of his or her organs—but rather what is being produced. The assertion of scientific authority enacted difference *from within* South-South cooperation. At times during that session with Dr. Roy, it seemed to me that Indian doctors performed a style of cooperation that shared a family resemblance with Prime Minister Nehru's pedagogical politics, discussed in chapter 1 as reenacting hierarchies among nations. The directionality of exchanges was turning African doctors and hospitals into a public in need of education. It was rendering them remote, in need of connectivity, and of being brought up in global circuits of biomedicine. One could sense a pattern that has been central to colonial rule, in which the imagination of a lack justified medical intervention, presented in the form of a gift. Representations of African hospitals as lacking and interchangeable also were common in discussions I had with PAN engineers and administrators. Without a doubt, the gift of PAN reshaped the relationships among connected peoples and places—within the clinic and beyond.

Global Enclosures

Critiques of global capitalism have often emphasized the key role of enclosures in producing new spatial formations while perpetuating economic dependence and underdevelopment. In global health in particular, *enclosures* refers to constrained spatial access to health resources, markets, and services. While they often result from deliberate policy decisions, such as the implementation of intellectual property laws that restrict access to essential medicines or the uneven allocation of resources, enclosures can also be the outcome of neoliberal attempts at global integration and inclusion. The notion of enclosure, however, is often accompanied by a conceptual ambiguity as it is used interchangeably with notions such as privatization, commodification, marketization, and exclusion, among other forms of deprivation—an ambiguity that, Sevilla-Buitrago notes, is "the result of an insufficient elucidation of enclosure's spatiality" (Sevilla-Buitrago 2015, 2). What are global enclosures made of? What is their material composition? What kind of work is required to maintain their spatial form, at least momentarily?

As mentioned in chapter 2, many social scientists have taken a materialist turn in the study of a variety of complex issues including climate change, ecological devastation, care work, digitalization, and global capital flows. Studies of infrastructure and technologies are no exception. While new materialisms are plural and not at all homogenous, they tend to share a conception of matter as lively and materialization as a "complex, pluralistic, relatively open process" (Coole and Frost 2010, 7). New materialisms challenge binaries between humans and nonhumans, undermining fantasies of mastery that have been central to modernist, anthropocentric accounts of science and technology. They also emphasize the primacy of movement over stasis, messiness over order, and constant transformation over enduring patterns and structurations. As such, they reject linear and deterministic conceptions of history, including of production, that can, for instance, be found in Marxism-inspired materialism.[33]

Sharing some of these orientations with new materialisms, although also influenced by ecological approaches, anthropologist Tim Ingold has built a strong case against the conception of place as a closed unit or a static location connected to other places by lines, themselves imagined as point-to-point connectors.[34] Ingold has instead argued for a conception of place entangled with and indeed emerging from living and moving lines. For Ingold, place is more than a spatial location. It is also events and continual processes of coming into being. Relations, then, do not connect discrete places, or nodes, as in a network. Rather, place is drawn out of interwoven lines of growth, as a knot in a meshwork. Interestingly, Ingold uses the example of the hub-and-spoke as a model that needs to be challenged because of the way it distinguishes the hub from the individuals it contains and from the lines connecting it to other hubs on the network.[35] The hub-and-spoke form, Ingold argues, is an ill representation of the actual processes of coming into being that animate life. However, Ingold's critique—with which I tend to agree—does not answer a different question of key importance as far as PAN is concerned: how can we account for the effective power of the hub-and-spoke form as it orders relations in concrete, material ways?

New materialist approaches to infrastructures and technologies can be useful in understanding how material things shape social, economic, and, in this case, medical practices. As I have suggested elsewhere with Tomás Sánchez Criado, however, new materialist emphasis on the vitality of matter and the ontologization of the interconnection between people, things, and environments often comes with a tendency to skim over historical processes of differentiation (Duclos and Sánchez Criado 2020). New materialisms have at times been charged with overlooking racialized and sexualized conditions of discursivity.[36] They also may appear to share in global capital's motto to simply "liberate the flows!" In other words, new materialist insistence on the immanence and indeterminacy of relations—including of growth—may conceal conditions of entrapment, leaving us ill equipped to examine the gestures of enclosures that constitute contemporary capitalism.

People, expertise, and things did not flow smoothly or emerge spontaneously in PAN. Instead, new connections emerged alongside enduring patterns of circulation and exclusion. Relations in PAN were also shaped by design. The hub-and-spoke model, it should be noted, was not solely a human construct, as it was indissociable from technological affordances, topographies, and other material considerations. Following the hub-and-spoke model, PAN was hierarchically and vertically nesting African hospitals within transnational pathways of expertise and treatment. PAN was simultaneously present in and removed from participating hospitals. It installed privatized, secured enclaves in public hospitals such as Black Lion and CHNU Fann. It essentially worked by avoiding hospital environments, which would have made the simultaneous implementation of a large network over dozens of countries an almost impossible endeavor. Derived from the model that guided the deployment of telemedicine within India, the hub-and-spoke model produced reservoirs of patients connected to yet partially insulated from global networks of biomedicine.

By connecting clinicians and patients, PAN brought them inside a spatial configuration that philosopher Peter Sloterdijk refers to as the "world interior of capital" (Sloterdijk 2013, i). The world interior produced by globalization, suggests Sloterdijk, consists of a complex network of interconnected and interdependent spaces that are constantly shifting and evolving. Sloterdijk compares this world interior to a series of archipelagos or islands, isolated yet connected through various channels of communication and exchange. The image of the archipelago provides a strong physical dimension to the spatial form: it gives it volume that, again, is often found lacking in discussions of enclosure. Perhaps no other thinker of modernity does that better than Sloterdijk. The writings of Sloterdijk are too multifaceted and wide ranging to be extensively discussed here. However, if we wanted to identify a theme underlying his ontological anthropology, we could suggest that it is concerned with the design of spaces in which life is being cared for and supported. To these spaces, which are at once material and symbolic, Sloterdijk gives the name "sphere."[37] For Sloterdijk, spheres—and indeed spaces—are not just abstract geometrical entities. They are not given. Rather, they are always *designed*.[38] Whether the earliest Paleolithic stone tools or the most sophisticated satellite technology, spheres are shaped by specific materials and technologies. They are also actively shaped by the models and concepts that humans use to understand and navigate them. Spheres can be physical structures, just like PAN's air-conditioned rooms, but they can also be conceptual structures like topological forms that regulate the circulation of people and things. In Sloterdijk's spheres, the modernist divide between materiality and design is dissolved away (Latour 2008, 2). Spheres are not static, watertight entities. Rather, they are fragile forms that emerge and collapse, expand and deflate, as things move across space and time.[39]

Like Ingold and new materialists, Sloterdijk thus proposes a relational ontology that, against any form of substantialism, emphasizes the centrality of being-with and in-betweenness. However, and this is a key distinction, as spatial formations, spheres are characterized by a sense of enclosure, containment, and separation. Just like for Geissler, discussed earlier in the chapter, globalization's enclosures for Sloterdijk are fragmented and partial. There is not much left of historical dreams of a full integration into a coherent, functional whole.[40] However, obviously not all humans inhabit the "world interior of capital" under the same conditions. An infrastructure such as PAN designed and connected indoor spaces: islands with semipermeable walls that, to some extent, isolated the interior from surrounding environments. Although the Rascom-QAF1R satellite assembled the continent under its material footprint, bodies and sites were differentially enveloped by the network. The artificial islands of PAN were no less conflicted or contradictory than "natural" islands or locations. They presented affordances and patterns that shaped the way human life was made visible and intervened upon at a distance. For patients like Aasiya, the circulation of expertise was not accompanied by better treatment. Following a hub-and-spoke model, patients had to travel to hubs—and, ultimately, to India. Aasiya could not afford to do so. If PAN had cultivated connections between African hospitals, who knows if Aasiya could have traveled to Mogadishu or, say, to neighboring Kenya for treatment?

To understand the spatiality of PAN, it is helpful to move beyond critical accounts of enclosure that tend to replicate (even as they oppose them) modernist conceptions of space, in which spaces are passive containers for human activity. By insisting on the indeterminacy and vitality of matter and things, new materialisms are most valuable here. However, it also seems important to supplement a new materialist emphasis on radical openness and permanent change with more sustained attention to the way spaces of movement can also become form. Addressing how movements of closure generate interior spaces helps give consistency to global capital without subsuming it under homogenizing globalism. The challenge, however, is to be able to think of vitality with stability, openness with enclosure, and indeterminacy with the antagonistic forces that effectively constitute the interior worlds of global capital.

4

THE EMPIRE OF SPECULATION

And to God the Almighty! Make my people sweat. Let their toil create many more Agnis that can annihilate evil. Let my country prosper in peace. Let my people live in harmony. Let me go to dust as a proud citizen of India, to rise again and rejoice its glory.

—A. P. J. Abdul Kalam (2003, 189)

India offers these networks to African countries. India is accompanying Senegal and the African Union in the conquest of tomorrow.

—Moustapha Guirassy, minister of communication and ICT, Senegal (cited in Ndong 2010; translation is mine)

"When we started, people said: 'Dr. Reddy, you're a crazy man.' Because we wanted to start a hospital here, they said: 'Are you crazy? Why are you doing all of this?' Nobody else thought that we could do it!" exclaimed Dr. Prathap Reddy, the founder of Apollo Hospitals, speaking in front of an audience gathered on the premise of Apollo's landmark hospital in Chennai. Every year on February 5, on the occasion of Founder's Day, the birthday of Dr. Prathap Reddy is celebrated. On that particular day, the atmosphere was festive. Several hundred employees and distinguished guests, including prominent members of the Indian political and business communities, were in attendance. "For the last decade, continued Reddy, 'we demonstrated to the world that we can deliver health care better than the best hospitals anywhere in the world. All of you have proved this. You have all done it! . . . There's nothing that we cannot do. This is not an ordinary thing. But we're used to do extraordinary things. It's spectacular!"

On that February morning in 2011, Dr. Reddy, who had already insisted with me during our private conversations on the need for Indian corporate hospitals to expand their footprint abroad, delivered a passionate call for a stronger, healthier, and more prosperous nation. According to him, Apollo's growth was an economic and moral project: making individual citizens healthier would contribute to India's economic prosperity and wealth. But even more importantly, Apollo's success story came with a deep sense of national pride. It nourished dreams of a new India, speculating on futures in which she would, at long last, stand on the top of the world:

[DR. REDDY]: In the last decade, the five world leaders have all visited India. Because of the promise that we are making! They want to be with us! There were days when you would say: "You're an Indian and 'hahahaha.'" But today, everybody's looking at us. That is what India is today. To keep our momentum, to go on and get on top of everything, we need healthy, happy people. People understand, they know the momentum coming from Apollo, and they say: "Wow, you have done so much for the country." We have made this country proud! By doing this, it's not just about being proud, we are building the new India that everybody is dreaming about. We are now helping the country to become a new India. Yes?

[AUDIENCE]: Yes!

[DR. REDDY]: And to be on the top of the world!

[AUDIENCE]: Yes!

On October 22, 2008, the Indian Space Research Organisation (ISRO) successfully launched its first unmanned lunar spacecraft from the Satish Dhawan Space Centre in Sriharikota, a peninsula in Southeast India. Launched using an Indian rocket—the Polar Satellite Launch Vehicle—the Chandrayaan-1 probe was to be placed in polar lunar orbit on November 8, 2008, to map the lunar surface for the next two years. Then, three weeks after the launch, on November 14, 2008, a small Moon Probe Impactor (MPI) was ejected from Chandrayaan-1. The MPI had several objectives. Equipped with a video imaging system, it had to take high-resolution pictures of the moon's surface before crashing in a deliberately uncontrolled way. The data received by the MPI confirmed the presence of water on the lunar soil and not only at the poles, as previously believed. "One Big Step for India, a Giant Leap for Mankind" was the headline of the *Times of India* following the publication of this discovery in the journal *Science* (Pieters et al. 2009).

On the evening of November 14, 2008, the man who came up with the idea for the MPI and insisted on making it a reality arrived at the ISRO command center on the outskirts of Bangalore just minutes before the MPI was to reach the moon. He came, like millions of Indians sitting in front of their television sets, to witness a historical moment. Twenty-five minutes after the MPI had left the orbital probe, the Indian flag crashed on the moon, painted on the four faces of the impactor. India had become the fourth country to put its flag on the moon—after the United States, the USSR, and Japan, but above all before China. It joined the ranks of global space powers. "That flag is a life. A national life. It should generate enthusiasm," President Kalam said after this important episode in the history of the Indian space program. The feat, Kalam insisted, would leave its mark on the imagination of the country's youth: "It has kindled a lot of interest in the young minds. When you ask children what is their dream, thousands want to walk on the moon. So I'm sure the Indian Space Research Organisation in fifteen years they will see to this that our astronauts walk the surface of the moon."[1]

If Kalam had his way, the first Indian would walk on the moon in 2025. Another would go to Mars in 2035. By 2050, human habitation would be extended to an economic complex integrating Earth, the moon, and Mars (Express News Service 2010). For Kalam, human development was inseparable from the emergence of a new relationship with outer space. Central to his work as a teacher and scientist was a speculation on the spatial, technological, and economic reconfigurations of the planetary future, in which India was called upon to play a leading role. For Kalam, investment in space technology, even though it was at times criticized in a country afflicted by massive poverty, was an investment in a new humanity and, above all, a new nation. Dreaming of the conquest of outer space, for the father of the Pan-African e-Network, was always also dreaming about the nation, prosperous and powerful.[2]

This chapter examines how PAN acted as an engine for economic and political speculation. I suggest that speculation in PAN was activated and channeled through the personae of Abdul Kalam as president, space scientist, and inspiration for the future of the nation. PAN was also grounded in and shaped by the material form of network infrastructure and the affordance of space technology in particular. This chapter takes seriously the efficacy of satellite form in producing distance.[3] The power of the satellite in PAN was just as performative as it was functional: it produced effects "as much through the desires people invest in it as through its ability to deliver predefined utilities" (Mazzarella 2010, 791). The same applied to President Kalam, whose charismatic persona fueled and channeled the entrepreneurial energies of the nation. Both Kalam and the satellite, I suggest, acted as mediums of expansion and unification. The network was a sort of echo chamber whose resonating effects contributed to identity building and strengthening. The (re)discovery of the nation and the global expansion of medicine and technology were feeding into one another. In understanding this relationship between identity and alterity, I further suggest that we must keep in mind that PAN was a gift that opened a space of indeterminacy and of speculation about future relations between giver and receiver, whether they be transactional, moral, or political.

Abdul Kalam: The Power of Dreams

For several weeks, my roommate Vijay had witnessed my interview-day preparation: revising the interview guide while having tea, uploading it to a USB drive to get it printed at a shop nearby, dressing up, and leaving early enough to leave some wiggle room for the unpredictable traffic in Delhi. Before I left, Vijay would often comment on my outfit, try to talk me into having one last cup of tea, and inquire about the places I was about the go to or the people I was about to meet. On one particular day, however, Vijay was stunned when I told him whom I was preparing to meet: after several months of emails, phone calls, and voicemail messages, I had an appointment with the former president of India Dr. Abdul Kalam. The meeting was set up in the late afternoon, at his 10 Rajaji Marg residence.[4] I did not know whether that was going to be a one-on-one discussion (it would) or how long it would last (half an hour). I also could not be sure I would actually meet Kalam. Would security let me in? I had been warned: Abdul Kalam was infamous for his last-minute cancellations. Despite his eighty years, he was a very busy man. Vijay could hardly believe it: His Canadian friend, who had left New Delhi several months earlier for Southern India, was coming back home not to spend his days in this or that hospital but to meet with the "people's president"? How was that even possible?[5]

Vijay's mix of astonishment and excitement was understandable. Before Kalam's passing in 2015, he was both an icon and an idol in India.[6] As an indication, in June 2012 *Outlook* magazine conducted a poll aimed at determining who was "The Greatest Indian after Gandhi." Names were preselected by a jury of scholars and celebrities who came up with their own rankings. *Outlook* then also conducted a nationwide poll by telephone and online. While only two of the twenty-eight members of the selected jury voted for Abdul Kalam (who was then no longer president) to be selected from the ten finalists, Kalam finished first in the telephone survey and second in the one carried out online, in front of figures such as Jawaharlal Nehru, Mother Teresa, Vallabhbhai Patel, and JRD Tata. Nearly 20 million people voted in the survey. The father of the Constitution of India and leader of the Dalits B. R. Ambedkar was ultimately proclaimed the winner, just in front of Abdul Kalam. Noting that Kalam had not made any original contributions to scientific or scholarly research, historian Ramachandra Guha (2012) lamented his high ranking, noting the discrepancy between the jury and popular perceptions of Kalam: "A. P. J. Kalam is a decent man, a man of integrity. He is undeniably a good Indian, but not a great Indian, still less (as the popular vote would have us believe) the second greatest Indian since Gandhi. Notably, the Net voters who ranked Kalam second also ranked Kamaladevi Chattopadhyay 50th or last. At the risk of sounding elitist, I have to say that in both cases the *aam admi* got it spectacularly wrong."[7]

According to Guha, then, the aam admi ("common man") was dramatically wrong in selecting Abdul Kalam as the greatest Indian after Gandhi. What is missing in Guha's account, however, is an understanding of how Kalam came to score so high. Kalam's popularity could not be reduced to a listing of scientific or technological achievements. In contrast to Guha's dismissal of aam admi's attachments as not grounded in historical facts, I much prefer the STS scholar Shiv Visvanathan's depiction of Kalam not as a mere scientist or political figure but rather as a performative spectacle in which people wanted to believe. Visvanathan is worth quoting at length:

> Look at the man, he is a performative spectacle. He oozes simplicity from every pore and with enough conviction to instill envy in a Dostoevskian idiot. His smile, childlike and saintly, made science appear accessible. He could have been a cult guru like Sri Sri Ravi Shankar holding forth on science as a solution to poverty and underdevelopment. He was literally official but could convey that "nothing official about it" look. Kalam's spirituality dissolved like sugar, sweetening Indian science. He created such a convincing front stage for science as deliverables that few thought of a backstage of doubt, ambiguity or failure. The ease of the man was inclusive. Children and heads of state both desperately wanted to believe in him. He blended all religions to create the scientist as the new missionary. For him, the transition from third world to first world, underdevelopment to development, could only be seen as a pilgrimage, a transformative act engineered by science. (Visvanathan 2015)

Kalam spoke to Indians in ways that resonated deeply with some of their most intimate, poignant political desires. Indians were *attached* to Kalam to the extent that he incarnated horizons of possibility and prospects of power. In a way reminiscent of Nehru, Kalam was an educator, hence his countless speeches to students and youth across the country. But perhaps his charisma had little to do with the content of the teachings themselves, which were not particularly original or entertaining. Rather, Indians who enjoyed Kalam appeared to *enjoy themselves in him*.[8] To his followers, the president offered an opportunity to participate in the revival of the nation. With and through Kalam, Indians could speculate about the future. The aam admi not only could dream but could dream *big*.

"Today, we have a GDP of 8.5 to 9.0%, it's nothing like a dream,"[9] Kalam explained to me when we met at 10 Rajaji Marg in New Delhi. "It is possible. We have to work hard. Our youth, they're on a mission! Major prosperity. We have to use their power and then definitively we are there. That's our dream." Kalam was a firm believer in the power of dreams but also in heavy labor and devotion to boost economic growth while building a strong, unified cultural identity. In Kalam's thinking, measures such as the GDP acted as a medium through which prophecy was sought: a new India was in the making.[10] Kalam was the life coach, the moral leader of the nation, aiming to give it back its confidence:

"We must get rid of our inferiority complex and defeat the defeatist spirit that plagues us" (Kalam and Pillai 2004, viii). For Kalam, the market replaced the state in the capacity to fulfill the developmentalist dream in India (Sundaram 2009, 14). Kalam called for the unleashing of creative, technoeconomic forces that had apparently been restricted for too long by a set of unfavorable historical conditions. Competitiveness became a national mission. It was the responsibility of every Indian to take charge of his or her life and realize his or her potential, itself entangled with the spirit of national renaissance or arrival. This vision of economic growth, however, is grounded in noneconomic elements and specifically in "hypernationalist dreams of a glorious ancient-modern future" (Kaur 2020, 16).

Central to Kalam's vision was technology. For Kalam, technology was a vital input toward the improvement of aam admi's living conditions. But it was also a vehicle for psychic and material strengthening. Although he often mentioned being inspired by Gandhi's teachings or by Buddhist philosophy (Acharya and Kalam 2009), Kalam's thinking remained fundamentally in line with Jawaharlal Nehru's modernist conception of development and progress, devoid of any criticism of scientific reason. Central to Kalam's rebranding of the nation as a land of science and expertise was information technology (IT). Kalam's IT dreams were not particularly original, however. Around the turn of the millennium, IT had indeed become the poster child for India's economic liberalization and increased participation in the global economy. The success stories of companies like Infosys and Wipro were the source of great national pride. Entrepreneurs like Dewang Mehta, Azim Premji, and Nandan Nilekani had become public stars. Unlike other sectors such as agriculture or manufacturing, the growth in the IT sector in India has been export led, establishing the country as a global powerhouse in the domain. Beyond economic measures, IT was to set an example: it was to show the world what India could do and nourish capitalist dreams of the nation brand. Former NASSCOM president Kiran Karnik thus described the branding process at work: "To make India and IT as synonymous as France and wine or Switzerland and watches" (cited in Einhorn 2002).

The branding of India as an ascending economic, scientific, and technological power often takes an ethnonationalist form. It mobilizes a mythological past and invokes a series of ethnocultural features. In the first decade of the millennium, there was a deluge of publications—essays, government documents, and so on—that actively branded India as a civilization with an ethnocultural predisposition for science and technology.[11] For example, two years before President Kalam announced PAN, the Planning Commission of the Government of India published a document calling for the awakening of "the dormant spirit of India," which located the country's potential for economic growth within its spiritual, historical, and cultural traditions: "Thus, it would be wrong to state that in 1947 India started to construct a modern nation from scratch. Rather, it began the process of rediscovering its rich cultural and spiritual values that had formed the foundation of India in the past. It is on this foundation that we seek to formulate our vision of India 2020" (Planning Commission 2002a, 2).

Similarly, Kalam's speeches and writings combined a desire to introduce India into the universal march of technological progress with the glory of the Indian civilizational heritage. To unleash the power within India, Kalam argued, she had to rediscover herself as a land of knowledge and technology.[12] For Kalam, such a moral and technological renaissance was also indissociable from strong cultural and political unity. In many ways, this is a recent version of a theme dear to Hindu reformers who sought, as early as the nineteenth century, to translate a sacred and grandiose history into the terms of colonial modernity. The colonial history of science and technology in India stages permanent tensions between on the one hand the domestication of the codes of a foreign power and on the other, claims to ethnocultural specificity. In *Another Reason*, Gyan Prakash (1999) finds in the origins of the Indian nationalist movement a translation "between the lines": the interstitial production of a fundamental difference from within the modernization process. Prakash shows how an Indian reformist elite produced under colonial rule a grammar of reform on the terrain of science that penetrated the depths of the Hindu cultural universe. Refusing the alien character of science and placing the origin of Reason in Vedic monism, Hindu reformers gave strength and direction to the emergence of an Indian modernity, allowing the rehabilitation of a nation lost under myths and superstitions. The ancient, then, does not take the form of a before but rather a contemporary form, which allows science to be introduced at the heart of the idea of the nation.[13]

The Hospital of the World

"India has been a hub of medical care for centuries. It has always been," explained Dr. S. K. Mishra when I visited the School of Telemedicine & Biomedical Informatics in SGPGIMS, Lucknow. It was thus only natural, he clarified, for the nation to redeem its status as a global medical hub. Dr. Mishra then proudly went on to explain how his hospital would soon be connected to the whole African continent—and how it already was connected to many neighboring South Asian countries to provide telemedicine services. At the time of my presence, network connectivity for PAN had just been installed and services were ready to start—two years after other Indian hospitals, however. Dr. Mishra cited technical issues to explain the delay. Perhaps, he also noted, the government had prioritized connecting private hospitals first. They were, after all, the ones who were primarily deemed to benefit from the network. But it remained, Dr. Mishra insisted, an honor to have been selected. It was not every day that one had the chance to be part of history in the making.[14]

Along with IT and satellite technology, medicine perhaps embodies better than any other field the contemporary reworking of India's ancient reputation for expertise. Telemedicine unites both. As explained in previous chapters, telemedicine in India was primarily developed as a means to reach new populations and expand markets across space. The largest Indian corporate hospital chains all do telemedicine. They also all participated in PAN. At the time PAN was launched, hospital chains all sought to make inroads into African markets. In addition to treating patients traveling from the continent, some provided various kinds of consultancy and management services to existing hospitals while others opened brand new hospitals or extended telemedicine services in Africa. Hospital managers and entrepreneurs I met in the course of this research were straightforward about the commercial motivation of their participation in PAN: the network would foster the transnational circulation of medical knowledge but also of data, patients, brands, and business cards. "It's like proving our existence. We are building a presence,"[15] explained a manager at the Narayana Hrudayalaya Health City in Bangalore when asked about his hospital's motivations for participating in the project. Through PAN, hospitals branded themselves as global hubs for medical care: "Caring for the World with World-Class Healthcare," as was suggested by Apollo Hospitals' slogan on the front page of a pamphlet distributed at the Ethio Health Exhibition in Addis Ababa.

By participating in PAN, medical entrepreneurs and managers speculated on future markets. PAN promised a presence and eventually profit, although uncertain and lying in the future. Speculation, however, was not restricted to commercial opportunity. PAN was not rational in any narrow economic or technological sense. It was a medium through which a certain idea of the nation was conjured into existence. A good illustration of this is to be found in the public and scientific debates surrounding the New Delhi metallo-beta-lactamase 1 (NDM-1) that was traced to India in 2010. NDM-1 is an enzyme that makes bacteria resistant to a broad range of antibiotics. NDM-1 was first identified in 2008 in a Swedish patient of Indian origin who traveled to New Delhi, where he acquired a urinary tract infection (Yong et al. 2009). However, the stir in India and abroad surrounding NDM-1 was triggered by the publication of a study in *Lancet Infectious Disease* on August 11, 2010—only a few months after PAN was launched—aimed at collecting more molecular, biological, and epidemiological data on NDM-1 (Kumarasamy et al. 2010). The paper, which presented NDM-1 as potentially a major global health problem, was coauthored by researchers from six institutes in India as well as others from the United Kingdom, Pakistan, Sweden, and Australia. Although the authors identified patients in India, Pakistan, and the United Kingdom, they also noted that "many of the UK NDM-1 positive patients had traveled to India or Pakistan within the past year, or had links with these countries" (Kumarasamy et al. 2010, 597). The paper specified that several of these patients had undergone surgery while visiting India and suggested that costs saved by these medical tourists would end up costing substantially more to their fellow citizens in the long term, as it would contribute to the spread of NDM-1 and in making it endemic worldwide.

Soon, the international press started covering the story of the "Indian superbug," emphasizing the country's high rate of infectious diseases, unchecked use of antibiotics, and unsafe drinking water supplies.[16] The inability of the Indian health care system to identify NDM-1 or treat patients adequately was also blamed for the spread of the "unbeatable" enzyme that could make all bacterial diseases resistant to antibiotics, to borrow the title from a *Daily Mail* article (Hope 2010). The blaming and shaming game associated with the coverage of NDM-1 triggered a massive response from the Indian government and industry. Indian ministers referred to the media and scientific reports about NDM-1 as unfair propaganda or conspiracy aimed at hurting Indian medical tourism. Government officials argued that such bacteria could be found anywhere, not only in India. Ms. K. Sujatha Rao, secretary of health and family welfare of the government of India, considered the article published by *Lancet Infectious Disease* to be "unscientific" and with an appearance of conflict of interest (due to funding from pharmaceutical companies) (Easton 2010). The director general of the Indian Council of Medical Research, V. M. Katoch, suggested the hype surrounding NDM-1 was deliberately manufactured to damage India's image as a medical tourism hub.[17]

The image in question had been carefully cultivated by the industry. In the years prior to the NDM-1 controversy, the safety of India as a destination for medical tourism was constantly questioned within the academic literature, media coverage, and political narratives in the global North. In response, India sought to brand itself as a safe destination for medical treatment. Indian hospitals secured international accreditations from organizations such as the Joint Commission International (JCI). In 2006, the Quality Council of India implemented the National Accreditation Board for Hospitals & Healthcare Providers (NABH) to monitor the safety of health care provided within Indian hospitals. The Eleventh Five-Year Plan (2007–12) of the Indian government stressed the importance of such certification to turn India into "a world-class destination" for medical tourism (Planning Commission 2008).

The debates surrounding NDM-1 underscored the enduring legacy of a colonial discourse picturing India as a land of filth, disease, and poverty. But it also made visible the strong nationalist sentiments underpinning the rise of India as a global center for medical care. In sharp contrast to the colonial imagination of filth and poverty, telemedicine came with the promise of a pure, uncontaminated clinical encounter. As was summarized in an article published by an online magazine from Madagascar, PAN made information travel instead of disease (Ramambazafy 2010). The network, the article suggested, offered a glimpse into the future of medical care: efficient, remote, and released from the affliction of physical travel and contamination. Telemedicine promised to carve out novel spatial configurations and enable hygienic postclinical medical care.

The strong affective investments in the NDM-1 scandal, just like in PAN, thus far exceeded commercial opportunity or economic rationality. It can be understood as an assertion of postcolonial autonomy and an opportunity to challenge the colonial roots of medicine and technology. However, while nationalist leaders emphasize the civilizational distinctiveness of indigenous expertise and science, the corporate hospitals that treat medical tourists mostly reproduce Western medical systems and models of neoliberal governance. So did PAN. Nevertheless, in both cases, scientific imagination contributed to defending *a certain idea* of the nation, helping India to become her true self, as President Kalam would have had it.

What is interesting in claims about India's past as a land of expertise is not whether such an idealized past ever existed. It is also not whether Indians actually want to return to it. What is fascinating is how nostalgic sentiments contribute to claiming autonomy and nurturing a sense of self in the present. Nostalgia, suggests the anthropologist Dominic Boyer, "always carried with it a politics of the future" (Boyer 2010, 25). This seems to apply pretty well to nostalgic discourse about ancient India, whether emphasizing medicine or technology. This discourse does not so much signal grief or obsession with the past. Rather, it is deployed to "mobilize a present- or future-oriented project of identification and belonging" (Boyer 2010, 20). The past, to borrow from Bharat Jayram Venkat, is not overcome "but constantly refurbished for a new age" (Venkat 2021, 5).

Millions of Lives

"Cheihh Gueye, a 9-year-old boy from Senegal, symbolizes the Indian government's engagement with the African continent better than anyone else," began an article published in *BusinessWorld* (BW Online Bureau 2012). Not too long ago, continued the article, Gueye was diagnosed with a life-threatening heart problem. Treating clinicians in Senegal recommended that he urgently needed to have a pacemaker implanted. However, they found the procedure too complex to handle locally. The young patient would need to be flown abroad in order to undergo surgery. This, indicated the article, was until an Indian doctor succeeded in instilling confidence in his Senegalese colleagues to carry out the procedure themselves. Dr. Ashutosh Marwah, a pediatric cardiologist associated with Fortis Escorts Heart Institute in New Delhi, offered his assistance. He would not do so in person, however, but rather from a distance of some ten thousand kilometers. Dr. Marwah thus recalled the events: "The doctors had never done this procedure on children before. They wanted the boy to be flown to India. But we convinced them that the patient may not survive the trip and needed immediate treatment. Under our guidance, the implant was carried out successfully and the boy is fine now" (BW Online Bureau 2012).

The surgery, the article moved on to explain, was part of a program apparently "doing wonders" in building relationships between India and Africa: the Pan-African e-Network. To provide evidence of the project's extraordinary scale, the article was accompanied by a map of the African continent showing the forty-eight countries covered by the network—the only nonconnected countries being Algeria, Angola, Equatorial Guinea, Morocco, South Africa, and Tunisia. The article specified that the network was launched in the context of a sharp intensification in bilateral trade, reaching $US60 billion between India and Africa in 2011. It highlighted the 23.6 percent annual growth in Indian exports to Africa and the increased contribution of the Indian state via lines of credit, capacity building, and soft skills development. The Pan-African e-Network, the article noted, was to serve as a "gateway into Africa"—an expression I heard time and again while researching PAN—for Indian companies, primarily in the medical sector. In doing so, the project was meant to build trust and affinity between business partners. Vimal Wakhlu, then chairman and managing director at TCIL, insisted that the project was "tremendously boosting the goodwill India enjoys with its African counterparts" (BW Online Bureau 2012). Or in the words of Ravi Bangar, joint secretary for East and South Africa at the Ministry of External Affairs of India, the network promoted an image of a benevolent Indian presence: "Are Indians liked in Africa? And the answer, he says, is yes" (BW Online Bureau 2012).

From its very beginnings, PAN benefited from exceptional public exposure. The inauguration ceremonies of its first two phases on February 26, 2009, and August 16, 2010, featured the participation of the minister of external affairs of India. Politicians and high-ranking government officials continuously visited the network's premises at TCIL and within participating hospitals. Photo opportunities were nearly as frequent as medical teleconsultations. President Kalam himself visited TCIL and gave a lecture that was broadcast through the network. These visits left traces. Images of Kalam—often taken while he visited—were frequently displayed within the offices and spaces of the network. PAN also received extensive media coverage in India but also in Africa and more globally.[18] The touring of reporters and journalists was frequent in PAN's studios. Media coverage advertised the network's feats. In such coverage, PAN's moral, commercial, and political claims met very little if any critical examination. In the words of TCIL's chairman Vimal Waklhu, PAN "was internationally acclaimed as the most successful project of its kind" (Wakhlu 2019). To some extent, the network was indeed celebrated. In 2010, for instance, it was awarded the Hermes Prize for Innovation for its contribution to the field of sustainable human development. This prize is awarded by the European Institute of Creative Strategies and Innovation, a think tank and research center that supports strategies for innovation. PAN was also adjudged among the "top 100 projects" of India in 2016, and TCIL was awarded the Skoch Renaissance Award in 2014.[19] PAN also found its way into official publications. The network featured prominently in the *Africa-India Framework for Enhanced Cooperation* adopted at the Second Africa-India Forum Summit in 2011. Such exposure added to an already long list of strategies to advertise the network, including commercial exhibitions, conferences, reports, and promotional materials.

I know of three films that were made about PAN: *Connecting Hearts: India's Pan African e-Network*,[20] *Connecting Hearts & Minds: India's PAN Africa Story*,[21] and *Bridging the Gap*.[22] All are short promotional films presenting the main components of the project. Funded by the Ministry of External Affairs of India, the films make bold statements about development, South-South cooperation, and technology. The films provide a comprehensive account of the network's architecture and of the services it provides. They feature engineers working in PAN's studios as well as fragments of CME sessions and teleconsultations. The films show images of TCIL headquarters and Indian hospitals including Fortis Healthcare, Apollo Hospitals, and the All India Institute of Medical Sciences (AIIMS). We can see doctors giving lectures and hear the testimonies of doctors, engineers, patients, and students explaining how the network touched them and impacted their life. The films also hint at the diplomatic life of PAN with segments from Abdul Kalam, interviews with diplomats, and recordings from its official inauguration in February 2009 by the minister of external affairs Pranab Mukherjee.[23]

The films feature images of networked wires, bytes circulating on digital highways, server rooms, engineers at work, youth on mobile phones, CT scans, ultramodern buildings, and a satellite looking down on both India and Africa from above. They stage an aesthetics of connectivity that associates electronic media with smooth communication, closeness, and a sense of humankind. "Ô human beings, why not you connect your hearts?" implores Kalam at the very end of *Connecting Hearts & Minds*. "The ocean connects us, the sky connects us, clouds connect us, [. . .] everything in the universe connects us," reads Kalam in the poem. Connectivity, President Kalam appears to suggest, goes to the very heart of human nature: to be in the world as a human is to be connected. For the connected human, the world is within reach. To be connected is to participate in the grand scheme of things in which bodies, spirits, hearts, and cosmic elements are harmoniously unified. Contemplating the effects of PAN, Kalam's poem can be read as a metaphysical statement: *everything* is connected.

The films perform a series of aesthetic and affective encounters with South-South relations. India and Africa, the narrator of *Connecting Hearts & Minds* suggests, dream together of a brighter future. PAN is "just the beginning, only a blueprint for the massive change that is to come." The films recount the story of an "Indian miracle" in the fields of health care and information technology, inciting viewers to imagine how it could serve as an inspiration for the future of the African continent. India, we hear in *Connecting Hearts*, can share with Africa a vision of growth and success in which technology is the key medium: "Technology has helped India script its growth story in the twenty-first century. Satellite, information and communication technologies have fueled a digital revolution that spans not just its own borders but aims to share its vision with Africa" (Radha and Shaw 2011).

On the one hand, the films do a fine job of challenging the hegemonic narrative according to which technology and expertise can travel only from the West toward the "technology-poor Global South" (Mavhunga 2017, 4). And indeed, as I have mentioned before, many of PAN's African actors appreciated the network as an alternative to such historical and deeply hierarchical pathways. On the other hand, however, in the films, technology and expertise are still assumed to be *imported* into Africa. The circulation appears unidirectional. There is no indication, in the films, of Africans being producers of knowledge: they are presented as recipients, not as agents driving scientific and technological innovation. They remain outside looking in. Here is a linear history of development, culminating with India's arrival on the global stage, celebrated for a worldwide audience.[24] In the words of Ravinder Kaur, "The spectacle of hope requires the "lacking" third world to be produced as a constitutive anteriority" (Kaur 2020, 16). The anteriority is to be found in India's past, with the failures and stagnations that preceded the miracle of economic reforms and "digital revolution." But anteriority is also assigned to Africa. If there was anything left from the Bandung Conference in the films, and indeed in PAN, it was the notion that India and emergent African nations were at different stages in their developmental journeys and that India was in a unique position to act as *vishwa guru*, which loosely translates from Sanskrit as "global or world teacher."[25]

The films about PAN systematically merge facts and fiction to the extent that they are practically indiscernible.[26] The films, for instance, overwhelm viewers with hardly commensurable images and figures. In *Bridging the Gap*, for instance, we can hear the TCIL chairman predict that "one million patients" will benefit from the telemedicine service. In *Connecting Hearts & Minds*, we can hear the narrator claim that the network is making an impact on an *immeasurable* number of lives. The narrator also suggests that PAN is a "modern, technological master-piece" that uses education and health care to "light up millions of lives" (Ministry of External Affairs 2012). Contrasting with the actual utilization of the network, such figures contribute to endowing PAN with a genuine power of fascination.

The numbers and figures invoked in the films are not meant to provide solid evidence of PAN's impact. PAN was not so much an experimental project as it was a speculative project. The distinction seems important. Anthropologists have done a fine job of pointing out how transnational experiments of many kinds have come to play key roles in the government of health care, including in contemporary Africa.[27] Studies have shown how these experiments have become subsumed under a logic of economic rationalization, the most widespread form of which is to be found in the search for measures of efficacy such as randomized controlled trials.[28] Imported from clinical trials, these techniques of accounting have migrated to other spheres of global health to ensure objectivity while claim-ing the moral authority of science. As explained in the introduction to this book, the dreams and promises of PAN were not mediated or made legible by such statistical technologies. There never was any controlled and systematic observa-tion and measurement. The futures that PAN conjured were simply not based on this kind of evidence. How could one ever quantify the inspirational power of dreams? How could one account for the futures they trace? PAN, in other words, was aimed at validation, not verification.[29] *Millions of lives.* The accuracy of such statements is not relevant. What is interesting here is not the objects of desire that PAN would be lacking: patients, markets, or any other particular end goal. It is how these objects are themselves the product of speculative desire.

Satellite Matter and Form

Hype, promise, and vision, argues Kaushik Sunder Rajan in his analysis of postge-nomic biotechnology, are primary drivers of a kind of valuation operating at levels that have little to do with tangible material indicators of present successful pro-ductivity (Sunder Rajan 2006). At such a level, value does not primarily depend on material production in the present but rather is driven by intangible abstractions: by "the felt possibility of *future* productivity or profit" (Sunder Rajan 2006, 18). The felt abstractions that compose promissory futuristic discourse, notes Sunder Rajan, cannot be opposed to reality: "Hype is reality, or at least constitutes the discursive grounds on which reality unfolds" (116). It is hard not to agree with a proposal to move beyond a cynical binary approach to hype and reality in which an "imagined" future would be opposed to a "material" present.[30] However, I suggest that making hype the discursive *grounds* on which reality unfolds is a steep price to pay as it risks asserting a problematic primacy of language. The question is: How does the "theologic mystique"[31] animating systems of valuation relate to the immanent world of things? Where are its powers coming from?

Promising, suggests Mike Fortun (2008) in his ethnography of genomics, generates futures in ways that carries an undecidability that is both constitutive and in excess of the present realities it folds back into. Because it is not possible to know if the promise in the future is empty or underwritten, promising is also always threatening. More importantly, notes Fortun, knowing about the emptiness of the promise would not in any way pre-empt its effects. In dialogue with Jacques Derrida but also with Shoshana Felman's writings on J. L. Austin and the speaking body, Fortun suggests that the scandal of promising does not so much lie in the manner it may be deceiving or failing promises—an infelicity that, for Austin, is constitutive of any promising. Rather, the scandal lies in the staging of a radical negativity in excess of any contradiction or opposition: a nonidentity that precedes and constitutes both subject and object. It seems to me that the play of otherness and difference here is not confined to the structure of the linguistic and the symbolic that we generally associate with promising. Just like finance, science is driven by affect as much as it is by rational cognition or experimentality. And because it works as an affective force that engages the body at a precognitive, nonconscious level, the limits of promising cannot be fixed by language. Why, then, do some technological objects generate excitement while others don't? What other material forces may be at stake?

Over the past decade or so, these questions have been raised with eloquence as part of the turn toward materiality that has largely shaped social science interest in infrastructures. As mentioned in previous chapters, new materialist approaches share a refusal to conceive of materials as inert substrate to which a certain meaning or significance would be attributed.[32] Infrastructures are not the outcome of the imposition of mental realities upon material ones. However, by overemphasizing the affective and prediscursive, new materialisms often— but not always—end up simply reversing the order between ground and the grounded, thus missing what happens not on the ground nor in abstract form but *in the middle*. As was laid out by Appel, Anand, and Gupta, the challenge is to examine how matter and form constitute each other without according primacy "either to the powers of human representation to account for material forms, or to the powers of materials in their imagined, ahistorical, elemental state to determine infrastructural forms" (Appel, Anand, and Gupta 2018, 25). However, I am less convinced that refusing to accord primacy to either materials or form necessarily leads to approaching matter as being "always caught up in meaning" (25) as the authors also seem to suggest. It all depends on what "being caught up in" entails. If it refers to the *exhaustion*, via discursive mediation, of the material's immanent potentials, the price again seems a steep one to pay. To claim that material potentials are historically mediated is not the same as refusing to grant material form any poetic or creative force of its own—a force that cannot be reduced to meaning any more than an artwork could, for instance. It does not violate the aesthetic autonomy of the infrastructural object to examine the conditions under which that autonomy is being produced.[33]

I suggest that central to PAN's magic lies the material affordance of the network and specifically of its satellite technology. As mentioned earlier, to connect African hospitals, PAN used bandwidth leased from RascomStar, a private company in which the primary investor is the Regional African Satellite Communication Organization (RASCOM). As described in chapter 2, the Rascom-QAF1R satellite used by PAN is entrenched within specific historical struggles and regional imaginaries. Launched into orbit in 2010, the satellite was developed to support regional autonomy and cooperation. Rascom-QAF1R was launched as a pan-African project in response to the Western domination of the satellite market. But beyond geopolitical interests and historical trajectories, the formal and material qualities of Rascom-QAF1R enable particular imaginations of the future: of the South, of the nation, and of the world to come. This is especially the case of satellite footprints. Covering the entire African continent, the footprint of Rascom-QAF1R provides more than a static map. It can "be thought about as a blueprint of regional future" (Parks 2012, 128).

The satellite is not an inert object to which meanings are attached and significance given.[34] It also is not pure material potentiality. In the satellite, materiality and form are mutually constitutive as they spur speculation on economic and political futures. This means taking seriously the power of forms to capture our attention and collectively enthrall us.[35] Attention to the poetic force of satellite technology is not new. Over fifty years ago, media theorist Marshall McLuhan was already probing the effects of satellite technology on human perception and imagination. Earth-orbiting satellites, McLuhan suggested, were not merely transmitting information. They were yielding a new perception of Earth as a human-made environment: no longer an invisible environment, Earth became an art form (McLuhan 1966, 93). The communication satellite, according to McLuhan, enables and constrains the way humans project themselves in space

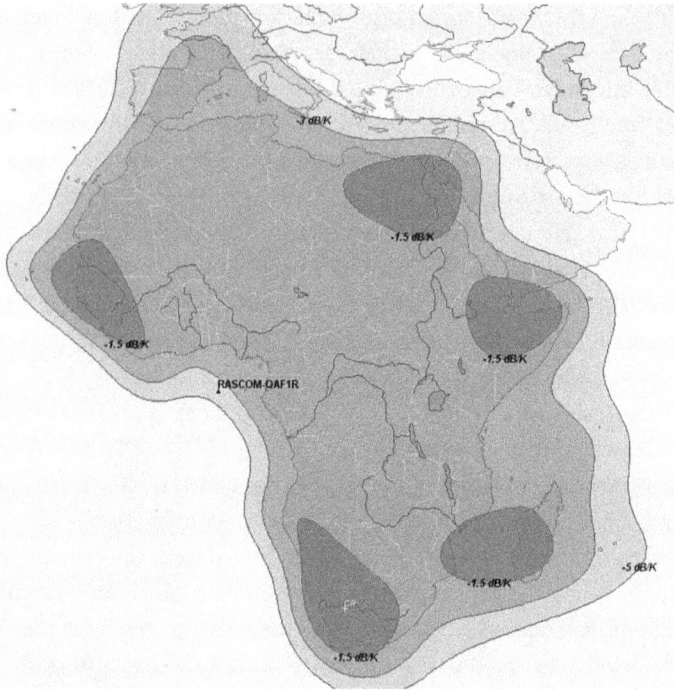

FIGURE 7.   Footprint of Rascom-QAF1R satellite C-band. Image used with kind permission of RascomStar.

and time. As medium, it introduces a "change of scale or pace or pattern" into human affairs (McLuhan 2003, 8). This does not happen at an abstract level. The satellite is rather experienced as a corporeal provocation, inducing significant sensorial effects and making things (in)visible that were previously not. The communication satellite, McLuhan notes, imposes a "new intensity of proximity," thus producing an "automatic response in all the organs of the body politic of mankind" (99). Form, for McLuhan, is not opposed to technology. Rather, form is technological, just as technology is in form.

Form matters in the sense that the satellite exerts a force at once engendering and shaping future possibilities. The form of the Rascom-QAF1R footprint is not imposed from the outside on the power of connectivity—it is immanent to it. The view from above afforded by the satellite, then, is performative in the sense that it does things in the world. The Pan-African e-Network holds together contending spatial forms that conjure different imaginations of the future: of the global South and indeed of a connected world.

This is true in at least two ways that could be framed as quasi-dialectical movements of expansion and enfolding. To start with, satellite technology invites fantasies of an endless expansion in space. Given its high level of mobility, satellite technology promises to bring bandwidth to hitherto unconnected hospitals, doctors, and patients. Bandwidth, suggested Kalam—himself a space scientist—in one of his many best-selling books, is a "demolisher of imbalances" (Kalam 2007, 175). It is deemed to be at once inspirational ("igniting minds," "inspiring thoughts") and aspirational (activating an upward movement both local and globally). Expansion comes with a disruptive and innovative intensification in exchange. PAN thus made us imagine a transnational sphere of exchange and intervention in which pools of patients are readily and remotely available. Through its practice of medicine at a distance, it exemplified a potential to circumvent old routes and infrastructures in the making of global biomedicine. The global health supply chain would never be the same again. The network performed a rupture between past configurations and new ones. It nourished the imagination of free, open, adaptable growth.

Second, as it intensifies expansion in space, the material form of the satellite also appears to enfold connected space and make it whole. Satellite communication stands as a metaphor for disembodiment, of placeless space. As the network expands through space, the roundness of Earth promises to transmute into some kind of unified totality or global embrace.[36] This relationship between space technology and Earth-as-form was superbly described by Peter Redfield in *Space in the Tropics*: "Space technology closed the sky again, bounded it from above and sealed it whole. Only then could the sky become fully modern in an active, technological sense, and only then could what lay beyond it become meaningful as space, a vast sea of darkness surrounding a blue and green point of human place. At last the world was one" (Redfield 2000, 123).[37] Here, satellite communication has little to do with information exchange or with expansion through space. Rather, it evokes a sense of communion and community: a sense of envelopment, which is not only technical or political but also aesthetic. This is what distance does: it suggests the internalization of outer space within the boundaries of a unified continent. Heterogenous, unbounded worlds are folded into a global, interior space. They are given a finite form. However, this comes at a cost: forms have the annoying habit of concealing the relations that are feeding into them.[38]

As was suggested by John Durham Peters, the modern notion of communication carries an imagery of magical, immediate communion that has long been in the making.[39] Communication, Peters argues, is concerned with the "transmission of immaterial forces or entities at a distance" (Peters 1999, 80). And the "medium"—the plural of which is "media"—is the mechanism for such contact between people via an invisible or elusive material connection.[40] Wireless communication such as radio or the satellite most obviously "boasts of action at a distance" (103) as it (re)activates a sense of immediacy and transparency in communication. With its "footprint" of continental reach from a celestial location, the satellite appears to be associated with divine or magical power (Peters 2015, 234).[41] Similarly, PAN was only ever solid when seen from above, from the satellite's vision of a distant, unified world.

To borrow cosmic and moral categories discussed earlier in the book, the material form of the satellite appears to invoke the spirit of cohesion of vasudhaiva kutumbakam. Under the enfolding grasp of its footprint, the whole world appears, indeed, as one family. Satellite technology thus appears as a medium of unification: technology holds the power to make the nation present to herself and to the world again.[42]

As a technological and entrepreneurial project, PAN was not only carried *in the name* of the nation (Irani 2019). Rather, the satellite gave form to the nation. Remember SITE and the early days of satellite technology for development in India, with its dynamics of close distance discussed in chapter 1: by reaching remote locations, the satellite embodied tension between unification and distant connections. Similarly, in a project like PAN, the nation envisioned itself differently and emboldened itself as a result of connections to distant peoples and places. By connecting in a new and wholesome way with the outside world, the national space was reconstrued and vibrating. It was its own sense of value that the hub animated and enlivened: it would become again, at long last, a hub of knowledge and care.

Passing Time

Krishnan[43] was in a bad mood when I arrived at the hospital. We hadn't known each other for very long, only a few days. However, on that morning, the engineer had a lot to say. He was in such a mood, he explained to me, because he had just learned some very disappointing news. Two months before, TCIL had announced the opening of four permanent positions for engineers. A few weeks later, Krishnan was called for an interview by the public company. This morning, he had learned that he was not selected. Of course, he knew that several other PAN engineers had also applied. But he really believed in his own chances to secure one of these jobs.

Krishnan was not only disappointed. He was angry. TCIL, he explained, ended up hiring only two engineers from PAN. The other two positions were filled with engineers from outside the company. Krishnan saw this as a form of betrayal. He kept emphasizing how long he had been waiting for this opportunity. Krishnan was adamant that he would now have to leave TCIL and find a job elsewhere. There was no indication that the state-owned company would be making any more permanent hires in the coming months, perhaps even years.

But, he explained, time was working against him. He was in his late twenties and still didn't have a permanent job. Krishnan wanted to get married. He was now discouraged. A good marriage, he insisted, depended entirely on the quality of the job: "I've wasted my life now."

The severity of the statement took me by surprise. But as the weeks went by, I came to better understand the reaction of Krishnan and most likely of other colleagues when they heard the same news. To understand Krishnan's reaction, it is important to know that there is a huge difference between contracts like the ones engineers had with PAN and the positions they applied for. PAN engineers were recruited as the network grew, mostly after responding to a job advertisement. The majority were men in their twenties with computer science or IT backgrounds in either college or university. They had generally not attended the country's elite institutions, such as the Indian Institutes of Technology (IITs), whose programs are extraordinarily hard to get into.[44] Beyond the hype that accompanied its rapid growth following the economic reforms of the 1990s, the IT sector was a cut-throat job market by the time PAN was launched in 2009.[45] Positions at multinational companies such as Google, Microsoft, Infosys, and Cisco were highly coveted and not easily accessible. The reason many engineers applied to work on PAN was straightforward: this was a job in the public sector for a company with a good reputation. TCIL also employed many engineers in permanent positions. These positions had little in common with the positions held by PAN's engineers. The salaries were much better, and by the end of an engineer's career, it would have tripled, perhaps even quadrupled. Above all, this was a permanent position in the Indian civil service that came with job security and benefits: "I could watch my belly grow," Krishnan caricatured. The civil service assured a certain quality of life. The engineers I spoke to wanted stable employment and thus financial security. They wanted the insurance plans and retirement funds that come with a government job. Others wanted to add that experience to their résumés. TCIL is a world-class company. Many engineers remain on PAN despite the monotonous, uninspiring work to get a good reference. Changing jobs frequently would not be a wise idea. It seemed better to wait it out.[46]

It is for all these reasons that dozens of engineers agreed to leave India, to go and work on the network in Africa. For many, this was no small thing. Several engineers, doctors, and managers working on PAN in India made it clear to me that they would never work in Africa themselves. They had a negative image of the continent. Their concerns were mostly related to food and security. An official of the Ministry of Foreign Affairs even suggested to me, "In some places, you do not even know if you will come back!"[47] To facilitate the recruitment of engineers for African sites, TCIL offered attractive working conditions. These engineers were, for example, paid twice as much as their colleagues in India as a remoteness premium. They also got forty-five days of paid vacation per year, which they spent in India.[48] The net result was that on the vast majority of PAN's African sites, TCIL engineers were of Indian origin. In this respect, the presence of Senegalese engineers at CHNU Fann in Dakar was an exception. Nevertheless, their motivation for participating in the project was similar to that of their Indian colleagues. In their midtwenties, both engineers were studying at NIIT-Senegal, the Senegalese division of the National Institute of Information Technology (NIIT), an Indian multinational corporation that specializes in "talent development" in the telecommunications sector. While working on PAN, they were completing master's degrees (MMS) in programming, specifically in software engineering. They were selected by NIIT to participate in PAN, partly because of their English-speaking skills. The two engineers' salaries were similar to those of their colleagues working in India—not those expatriated in Africa. They also did not get paid vacation time. While the two engineers did not associate their participation in PAN directly with possible socioeconomic advancement as their Indian colleagues did, they emphasized that it was a good experience to add to their résumés. They were participating in a transnational project with high visibility. In addition to their degrees from an international institution (NIIT), work experience in a multinational company such as TCIL was a valuable asset for young IT experts about to enter the job market.

For the engineers working on the network, PAN could be a source of great hope. Because of the scope and prestige of the network, PAN was imagined as a gateway to other professional horizons. Some engineers still speak of their work and travels with great pride, even with an element of embellishment. Engineer Manish Dhameja used PAN to collect world records and receive awards both in India and abroad—including in Madagascar, where he was posted for many years. He now apparently holds seven world records, including one for achieving the most degrees under thirty years of age: seven master's degrees, two bachelor's degrees, and six certificates. Manish has also become famous in India for his vast collection of rare coins, partly collected via his own travels and those of TCIL colleagues, which earned him a place on various lists of world records, including Guinness World Records.[49] PAN, for him, opened up a world of opportunities. The network, for him and others, became a central story in a much broader narrative in which public exposure, personal fulfillment, national pride, transnational journeys, and speculation on the future were deeply entangled.

Most PAN engineers, however, did not set any world records. Just like Krishnan, they thought of themselves as underemployed. Often highly qualified (with BTechs or master's degrees), they considered their work on PAN to be quite boring, repetitive, and not making the best of their skills. Many would also have preferred working closer to home. For these overqualified Indian engineers, being hired by an Indian government company to work on such a prestigious state project hinted at the possibility of a highly coveted future position: a government job. Krishnan and his fellow engineers remained in limbo, which was indissociable from the speculative logic of PAN: The economy was ready to take off. The nation was about to rediscover its true self. They only had to hang in there. Waiting, however, was obviously ridden with the anxiety of not making it into the world of global capital and slipping back into the waiting room of history.[50] There was no certainty for engineers, and indeed for any of PAN's actors, of a return on their investment, whether it be affective, financial, or otherwise.

The Project Is a Gift Is a Project

PAN, this chapter has suggested, was a project shaped out of heterogenous expectations and affective investments. The promises of telemedicine in India were embedded into its design: first, a socialist vision of development, and more recently, the project to integrate remote locations into a unified landscape of medical expertise, examined in chapter 1. So was the historical promise of the Rascom-QAF1's satellite, which was to foster regional autonomy and was now "given back" to Africa as part of a project aimed at transnational market expansion. As examined in the previous section, the network engineers had expectations of their own. They spent peak working years doing rather repetitive, uninspiring work expecting future job security. Although they were financially compensated for their clinical work on PAN, for many Indian doctors PAN was also much more than a mere economic transaction. Sharing their expertise and mentoring colleagues came with a sense of duty and pride. Entrepreneurs imagined the project as part of a broader vitalism of growth whose signs they detected in India's skyrocketing GDP annual growth rates, which had just reached the magical number of 10 percent in 2010. They were on a mission. For politicians and diplomats touring the network's studios with visitors or presenting it on stages worldwide, the network came with a joy of giving in public. All these affective projects, enfolded into PAN, were not rational in a narrow economic sense. They were autonomous from its commercial or technical functions.

In this chapter, I have tried to show that the affective investments in PAN were indissociable from the logics of speculation in global, capitalist India. In the following pages, my aim is to further explore the temporality of PAN by emphasizing its status as a gift. It seems important to keep in mind the question President Kalam identified when we met as the impetus that led to the creation of PAN: what can India give to the world? Gifts have long been a focus of anthropological inquiry.[51] In his seminal work, *Essai sur le don*, Marcel Mauss proposed foundational theories on gift-exchange systems that still remain the primary inspiration for anthropological studies of the gift (Mauss [2002] 1925). In the following decades, an impressive amount of scholarly work has documented the rules of gifting, receiving, and returning gifts in specific societies. Anthropologists have examined how gift exchange has been, in various forms and across cultures, instrumental in fostering and strengthening social ties, including through a sense of indebtedness. Gift exchange has often been studied to complicate and hopefully move beyond the Western notion of *Homo economicus*, with its assumptions that all human behavior can be explained in terms of economic rationality. Through studies of gift exchange, anthropologists have explored the relationship between persons and material objects.

Perhaps above everything else, anthropologists have located obligation as a driving force of gift exchange and thus sought to understand its mechanisms. What is it, as Mauss famously asked, that compels the recipient to return a gift? Studies of the gift have emphasized the principle of reciprocity as a social obligation that creates a lasting bond between giver and receiver. Gift scholarship has also tirelessly debated Mauss's own answer to the question of reciprocity—namely, the suggestion that gifts carry with them something of the giver's identity, often discussed in terms of the *spirit* of the gift, that elicits a return gift.

Gifts, the anthropologist Guido Sprenger recently argued, create futures that remain indeterminate (Sprenger et al. 2023). To emphasize such an indeterminacy, Sprenger replaces "obligation" with the notion of "expectation" as the grounding concept in gift exchange. When engaging in gift exchange, according to Sprenger, actors expect something to happen, but the range of expectations is extraordinarily wide: "The futures that the gift brings into being contain a variety of—often almost equally—likely possibilities, including nonreturn" (76). The form taken by reciprocity, and indeed the very presumption of reciprocity, shall not be taken for granted. To give is to expect in rather indeterminate ways. It includes an element of speculation. Thus, thinking of gift exchange in terms of expectation draws attention to the future possibilities the gift creates. The gift can then be understood as "a 'project' in the original sense of 'to be thrown ahead'" (77) toward uncertain futures.

I have found this foregrounding of expectation to be helpful in trying to understand the temporality of PAN as a gift. As its full name suggests, the Pan-African e-Network Project always was a *project*. The futures created by PAN always were and remain unspecified. There always was a possibility that PAN would remain unreciprocated. There was no explicit demand or agreement about an immediate or future return. Expectations about a return were not formalized in legal and financial terms. Despite their insistence on the high value of the gift, however, PAN actors could only speculate on the likelihood of reciprocation and the nature of the return. What would a counter-gift be? Of course, in India, there were expectations of future market expansion, hence the discourse of a win-win South-South cooperation. But when, where, and to what extent exactly would this happen? International awards, films, and the attention of journalists—or of an ethnographer such as myself—also came with a sense of gratification: They communicated regard. But was this recognition or self-aggrandizement really sufficient to be considered a form of reciprocity?

On the one hand, then, the status of PAN as a gift contributed to making it into a project. The shared future it opened onto was largely uncertain. On the other hand, however, obligation could also not be fully discarded. Even though PAN was not used at full capacity by its recipients, as the next chapter suggests, they also could not freely dispose of it. There was an obligation to care for it in one way or another. Then, the future that the gift works on does not emerge from scratch but rather "from the past, insofar as expectations are generated by experience" (Sprenger et al. 2023, 78). This applies to PAN, which very much emerged from complicated, regional histories of cooperation and market exchange. PAN, again, did not come out of a humanitarian aid program. And the commercial and political expectations of its actors materialized in the network's design in such ways that certain futures appeared more probable than others. Power dynamics and asymmetric relations shaped or stabilized identities between trade partners and giver and receiver. They gave the network its topology and spatial form. Then the question is: In PAN, did expectations open up or narrow the field of possibility?[52] The next chapter provides fragments of a response to this tricky question. It does so by giving special attention to the issue of poor utilization of the network. As the chapter suggests, in the implementation of PAN, new delays were constantly introduced and futures postponed. PAN was the site of a constant struggle between a universalist vision of the future and the actual ambiguities and elusiveness of the futures expected in the present. For better and for worse, the map never really coincided with the territory. In the meantime, all one could do was wait.

MAPS AND TERRITORIES

Model-thinking—always in the normative sense of
"model"—is empire thinking, be it occidental or oriental.

—Eduardo Viveiros de Castro (2019, S303)

"Good morning to all, I am Shyamala Das, consultant urologist from Chennai,"
announced Dr. Das. "In today's CME program, I'm going to talk to you about
overactive bladder," continued the urologist from Apollo Hospital. After a quick
pause, Dr. Das looked at the computer to her right, where the PowerPoint presentation she had designed for the occasion appeared. Dr. Das then began her
lecture. She spoke slowly, taking short pauses between sentences and emphasizing important terms. For over half an hour, the urologist presented epidemiological data and discussed the etiology of an overactive bladder. She addressed the
stigma associated with the condition and its underdiagnosis. Dr. Das also provided guidelines for clinical diagnosis, medical history, and physical examination.
She reviewed various tests that can be done on a patient and talked about similar
diagnoses. She presented clinical cases with ample details. Dr. Das also introduced treatment options ranging from changes in diet to medication, behavioral
therapy, and pelvic floor exercises.

Dr. Das's explanations were clear and supported by slides presenting lists, defi-
nitions, graphs, tables, and images. She spoke slowly, and it was easy to understand
what she was saying. In her forties, Dr. Das had been practicing at Apollo Hospital
for a few years. Before that, she trained and worked for over a decade in the United
Kingdom. A frequent speaker at international meetings and conferences, Dr. Das
was accustomed to teaching and speaking in front of an audience. She arrived at
the PAN offices half an hour before her scheduled presentation, which she had
prepared with great care—as did most of her colleagues. A question, however, was
left unanswered: would anyone be listening to what she had to say?

As with every session, Ashoka, the TCIL engineer at Apollo, had checked beforehand with every PAN engineer to see if there were any audiences in their respective hospitals. This was done by chatting in Virtual Tele-Ed, the software used for CME sessions. "Any attendance?" he would simply ask. Most of the time, if no one was there, engineers did not bother replying. Others would answer, "Nil." On the day of Dr. Das's lecture, however, the answer of the engineer stationed at the Medical Institute of Madagascar (IIM) in Antananaviro attracted our attention: "10–15 attendance." Other than the IIM, only one person would attend the conference, from the Libyan Board of Medical Specialties in Tripoli. A few minutes later, Dr. Das thus faced a large flat screen in which a dozen people could be seen sitting at desks set up in what looked like a classroom (but was part of the PAN studios at IIM). Since IIM had the only audience worth mentioning, Ashoka had opened only one window in Virtual Tele-Ed. Had there been another audience elsewhere, he would have split the screen into a few windows. This way, Dr. Das would see only the audience gathered in the IIM.

Along with teleconsultations, CME sessions were a primary service provided by PAN. From Monday to Friday, except for public holidays (the number of which in India cannot be underestimated), three or four sessions similar to the one described above were broadcast live in every hospital connected to PAN. The lectures took place from 2:30 to 3:30 p.m., 3:40 to 4:40 p.m., 4:50 to 5:50 p.m., and sometimes from 6:00 to 7:00 p.m., India Standard Time (IST). PAN was able to offer so many sessions simply because of the number of participating hospitals: each of the twelve Indian hospitals offered six sessions per month. Over the course of a year, several hundred hours of continuing medical education (CME) were therefore delivered through the network.[1] At CHNU Fann, CME sessions are held from 9:00 a.m. to 12:30 or 1:30 p.m., GMT. At Fann, however, sessions had generally little in common with the lecture described above, given by Dr. Das, with good and responsive attendance. Rather, CME sessions took place in an atmosphere combining the indifference of routine and the strangeness of an ignored presence. Every morning, Jean-Louis and Sada would set up the equipment for the sessions. A few moments later, the broadcasting of the lectures started on the wall of the PAN room. On the screen, we could see lecturers talking and gesticulating. Slides would come on and off. The sound was generally turned off, as there was no one in attendance. The room was filled with empty chairs. The engineers kept themselves busy working on some other things, and so did I. On the wall, the speakers came and went—ghostly presences appearing and vanishing in silence.[2]

Indian doctors were generally easy to persuade to be speakers in PAN. It was paid work.[3] More importantly, many were intrigued by the experience. Before the session, there often was a sense of excitement, especially when the speaker was lecturing for the first time over the network. Speakers generally took their time to speak slowly and prepare slides for their lecture. There was a concern for a job well done. However, lecturing on the network was not always an easy experience. Lecturers were often presenting to very few if any people in attendance. While African hospitals without any attendance would generally leave the camera off in order not to stream images of empty chairs, it was not always the case.[4] As a result, speakers often had to virtually speak in front of empty rooms.[5] This situation affected the morale of the speakers. Several mentioned to me that they found the experience of speaking in front of low attendance to be tedious. For example, this rheumatologist from Apollo: "The camera is not a problem, but with no audience, it feels special. The ambiance is not good."[6]

"We are giving talks to tables and chairs," expressed Dr. Ganapathy, an Indian doctor and manager discussing his participation in PAN. However, low attendance at CME sessions was only one component of the poor utilization of the network. Two years after the network was launched, only a few hundred medical teleconsultations had been conducted, which remains very low when taking into consideration the huge expenditure that PAN was. Again in the words of Dr. Ganapathy, commenting on the gap between what his hospital could provide and the small number of requests from African hospitals, "The utilization is way down. I have the capacity to provide specialists for fifty teleconsultations *a day*! In twenty-five different specialties. You name it and I can get any specialist here within one hour."[7] Poor utilization was no secret; TCIL managers always acknowledged it as a problem. The majority of the project's actors I met during this research agreed on one point: there was a gap between the projected and the tangible impact of PAN, and it was mainly the consequence of the network not being used enough. Poor utilization was upsetting. It embarrassed doctors lecturing in front of empty seats. It annoyed managers whose hospitals were seldom requested to provide teleconsultations.

Recent publications about medical interventions in sub-Saharan Africa, notes the medical anthropologist Nolwazi Mkhwanazi, tend to put forward a single story of medicine, health, and health-seeking behavior (Mkhwanazi 2016). This dominant story, Mkhwanazi tells us, is primarily concerned with the *unpredictability* of biomedical technologies and interventions—mostly designed and funded in the Global North—in local settings. The story unfolds in three parts. First, it is a story about the state's poor involvement in the provision of health, specifically about structural inequality and poverty and how they affect access to health care. Second, the story stages suspicion and distrust, whether between Africans and foreigners (mostly from former colonial powers), between Africans and the state, or among Africans. The third component of the single story, Mkhwanazi explains, often connects the first two parts by underlining "the creative crafting of knowledge, meaning, and action" (197) at the local level. In doing so, the story insists, Africans are not passive victims of failed interventions. Rather, they are active in finding solutions—for example working tirelessly in difficult conditions or improvising with the little resources available.[8]

It always seemed to me that the story of PAN, and of its poor utilization in particular, did not fit the "single story" recounted by Mkhwanazi. To begin with, the story of PAN is not primarily about the creative fashioning of knowledge, meaning, and action in response to scarce resources. It is not a story about improvisation or DIY medicine and technology. PAN certainly does not feature passive African actors waiting to receive health care or technology. And I also do not mean to suggest that imaginative practices of care did not take place. Doctors, engineers, and managers certainly did improvise. However, in the everyday life of PAN, the creativity of its actors—including the labor they put into building connections—was practically constrained by the structuring of the network as an infrastructural form. As the following pages will show, this took many different forms. Some gave up, ignored, or refused to participate in the project. Equipment never got dispatched to some hospitals or did not make it through customs. Expertise got lost in translation, becoming useless or unintelligible. In PAN's story, although they never were the passive recipients of expertise, African actors were not much involved in the design and implementation of the network. Their concerns and opinions were later acknowledged, but the network infrastructure already appeared too big and not flexible enough to accommodate them. So, to borrow once more from Mkhwanazi, if this is not a story about the unpredictability of technological intervention, then what is the story here? I suggest that the story of PAN is about dreams and assumptions of total control and seamless expansion, which are simultaneously underpinning and undermining PAN—thus contributing to the poor utilization of its medical services.[9] It is a story about the practical consequences of distancing and spatial ordering.

In the following pages, I start by providing an overview of the primary factors—effective and imagined—that have been frequently mentioned by PAN's actors to explain its relatively poor utilization. I then move on to present what, based on my ethnographic inquiries into PAN, can be seen as the main organizational factors underlying or even going against the individual factors identified. PAN, I suggest, tirelessly attempted to bend material realities—of biomedicine but also of networking, labor, and commerce—to be in line with powerful imaginaries at work in dreams of scale. The desire for rapid, seamless expansion and speculative futures undermined the conditions for PAN's existence in the present as it compromised the messy mediation work required for a project like PAN to be viable. Low utilization emerged as the flip side of dreams of total control, operationalized by a hub-and-spoke model: to leave intact the image of the network, its corporeality had to be sacrificed. As such, it destabilized binary modes of thinking as they crystallized opposition between design and implementation, network form and infrastructure, and map and territory.[10]

A Lack of Knowledge

For a majority of Indian actors involved in PAN's telemedicine services, a generalized lack of awareness about the network was considered the primary factor impeding its better utilization. Whether at TCIL, the Ministry of External Affairs, or in Indian hospitals, lack of awareness was the prime suspect. Service providers lamented the absence of efficient communication channels with potential users. Lack of awareness was not limited to the circulation of information about the *existence* of the project. According to Indian stakeholders, it also came with a need to better educate doctors about the benefits of its services. A senior executive at Fortis Escorts Heart Institute in New Delhi commented, "It's a great tool. But they've not been able to *sell* it to the people who would use it. I think it requires two hands to clap. So simply providing the solution is not enough."[11] Dr. Ganapathy, pioneer of telemedicine at Apollo Hospitals, was straightforward when we discussed this in 2011: "The Government of India has spent 250 million dollars or something like this already, but they have not spent any money on creating awareness! Unfortunately, 'marketing' is a dirty word. 'Lobbying,' 'marketing,' whatever you call it. . . . But for several reasons, lack of awareness is there unless you're on the radio, on television, you meet people, you invite doctors from India to go and visit all these hospitals, etc. This is hardly done."[12]

Overall, there is a general sense of a need to convince African doctors to use the network by providing them with more information. "A lack of awareness is there. People have to understand what are the advantages of telemedicine,"[13] noted a senior manager at Fortis Noida, another participating hospital. "We want to persuade them!" a senior official at the Ministry of External Affairs expressed without hiding a sense of exasperation.[14] In response to the situation, the Ministry of External Affairs and TCIL implemented different initiatives to try to persuade their African counterparts. Workshops were held in New Delhi, bringing together over sixty hospital managers, equipment suppliers, and national coordinators for the project.[15] J. L. Kachroo, project director for TCIL in Africa, noted, "We're trying to sell it but it takes time. It's a new network. There is resistance from the local side but this has to be worked on. We are trying to make people understand the usefulness of teleconsultations in particular. As far as TCIL is concerned, we have provided the network. It's in place. About its usage, it is for the local authorities to inculcate in the minds of the doctors."[16]

At the heart of PAN was a desire to incite clinicians to make teleconsultations part of their everyday clinical practice. The project was based on the premise that it was in the interests of both doctors and patients to call upon the expertise of Indian medical specialists. Consequently, connecting to the network was considered to be a rational, logical choice and even a form of professional responsibility. Expectations related to the project thus relied on the idea that potential users shared this vision of their own and their patients' interests. Convince people. Inculcate in their minds. Make them understand. This was the kind of discourse I heard over and over again when the time came to explain why most hospitals barely used PAN's telemedicine services. The aim here was not simply to make doctors aware of PAN's existence but really to coax them to use it by raising awareness of its benefits. In this regard, some Indian stakeholders lamented the absence of African telemedicine "champions" who could help promote PAN in their respective countries. By contrast, hospital managers I met in Africa pointed out that they were not the ones who had come up with the idea of the network. They also were not the ones who had designed it this way.

Failure at persuasion sometimes shifted to blaming. When the time came to make sense of the lack of enthusiasm of African doctors regarding PAN, their egos were often identified as culprits. A senior official at the African Union Commission explained, "First, doctors have a big ego. They think they have nothing to learn from others."[17] This ego, which apparently prevented doctors from enjoying the benefits of networks, was frequently mentioned in discussions on utilization with the project's managers. "They do not like to be told what to do,"[18] commented J. L. Kachroo. Another senior official at TCIL explained, "Here again the question of the ego of the doctor comes into the picture. Whether you would like this patient to be shown to an Indian doctor. You know, doctors are having this kind of feeling that 'my patient might feel that I'm not competent enough and that's why I'm showing to somebody else.' Whereas it should be the other way around. My value, in regard to my patient, will increase if I facilitate his better treatment by bringing him to this center and showing him to another specialist. So my patient might feel that 'look my doctor is very good! He's doing his best. But he's going beyond that! For my betterment!'"[19]

Doctors who refused to integrate the network into their clinical practices were thus presented as compromising PAN's mission to improve the medical care of their patients. This was often framed as a form of resistance to change.[20] Once again, an official at the African Union Commission explained, "It is threatening doctors. Maybe it would replace them. This is an issue of resistance to change."[21] Resistance to change was often viewed as a form of conservatism. Some also believed that the provision of free services might raise suspicion. Suggestions to offer African doctors financial incentives to participate or to make participation mandatory were common. Others cited vague cultural or behavioral factors such as a lack of entrepreneurship or discipline or perceived laziness. Overall, then, negative attitudes toward the network were often interpreted as a form of resistance to be overcome. Doctors had to be educated about the benefits of their participation in the project. Resonant with (post)colonial forms of accusation and patronizing, the blaming of PAN's poor utilization on the recalcitrance of African doctors made them, as nonparticipants, into an index of otherness. It suggested that they did not know (yet) what was best for them and their patients.[22] But ultimately, and this is critical, most Indian actors of PAN appeared convinced this lack of awareness, or recalcitrance, would eventually be overcome. The moment PAN would fulfill the expectations they placed into it was always only *delayed*. As mentioned in the introduction to the book, this notion of delayed fulfillment explained away the issue of low utilization, which was always considered provisional. African doctors would *eventually* be persuaded. It was always merely a matter of time.

Challenging both the blaming of doctors and the related inevitability of a persuasion to come, discussions with African doctors revealed that their reluctance to use the network was not due to a resistance to change or to telemedicine itself. Rather, African doctors expressed specific concerns about how the network impacted clinical work. They explained that while teleconsultations were occasionally helpful, they could also create a sense of helplessness. At times, they emphasized, there was a significant disparity between the expertise provided through the network and the local capabilities for diagnosis or treatment. A neurologist at CHNU Fann in Dakar explained, "Indian specialists have access to diagnostic equipment that we do not have here. Sometimes they might suggest: 'You have to do this.' But we can't! Access to medical care is very limited, for technological and economic reasons. Often patients can't afford tests or treatments. Sometimes we already know what we should do in the best-case scenario, but we can't do it. In these cases, teleconsultations can become very frustrating. These are the limits of the network."[23]

As previous chapters have shown, medical expertise was not merely circulating on the network. To have any therapeutic relevance, it also had to be translated (or adapted, mediated) in many ways. Distance between vision and practical conditions, between the promise of delocalization and the embeddedness of medicine, ran through the experience of PAN, not as an occasional gap but as a key feature of the network. African doctors were not equipped to bridge this gap. From the perspective of African doctors, their reluctance to use the network was not viewed as resistance to change but rather as a struggle with the difficulties of mediating between different medical worlds, a process that could be time consuming and impact their practice. Although many African doctors acknowledged that the network could offer certain benefits, it also induced feelings of helplessness and irritation, contributing to their hesitancy in using it.

Lost in Translation

Communication over the network was often messy and complicated. To begin with, PAN was predominantly an English-speaking environment. Teleconsultations and CME sessions were conducted exclusively in English, and the website, working documents, workshops, and formal activities related to the project were also only in English. However, English is not the mother tongue of many (if any at all) of the network's participants, who speak languages such as Hindi, Tamil, Punjabi, Wolof, Arabic, and Amharic. While the use of English as a common language helped to expand the network across various countries with different linguistic backgrounds, standardizing communication, many participants felt it was also a barrier to greater use of the network. Doctors who were not proficient in English were hesitant to request medical teleconsultations, and language barriers affected attendance at CME sessions. Many African doctors reported having difficulty understanding their Indian colleagues during lectures, a challenge particularly evident at CHNU Fann, where most doctors speak French but are not accustomed to working in English. Communication was further complicated by strong regional accents. As was noted by a cardiologist, "Language is a primary cause of low utilization. Doctors are not comfortable using the network."[24]

Take again the example of the CME lecture given by Dr. Das from Apollo Hospital. As was sometimes the case with CME sessions with an audience, the lecture was followed by a few questions. This did not come as a surprise: during the urologist's presentation, the audience listened carefully. This was not always the case. Just a few days earlier, for example, I had attended a session during which members of the audience did not pay much attention to the lecture, and we could see them talking and laughing with each other on the screen. This day, in contrast, the audience showed obvious interest. Some took notes, and others nodded or smiled. When the time came for the Q&A, however, audience members struggled to speak in English. Like in many other sites connected to PAN, English is not frequently spoken by Malagasy doctors. Most can follow a presentation and understand most of the content, but asking questions is a different story. At the end of Dr. Das's lecture, someone—most likely a doctor, although she did not introduce herself—aimed to ask a question. However, she struggled to do so. As it became evident that Dr. Das did not understand the question, Ashoka prompted me to please join the urologist in the studio. The audience was told that someone would now be doing some translation work. They could hear my voice but not see me, since I was sitting at the back of the room.[25] "What are the side effects of the treatment on the skin?" the woman in the audience asked once again, now in French. I turned to Dr. Das with a translated version of the question. The urologist answered, still looking at the camera, after which I translated her reply. The same audience member then inquired if there was an equivalent medication that could be as effective. Dr. Das began to list several types of anticholinergic drugs before turning to me: "Ask them what is available, from the slides that I have shown them. Is oxybutynin available?" I did so, but no one answered the question. Dr. Das insisted, "Ask her again. Is oxybutynin available?" Just as I asked again, there was an audio issue. We could not hear the audience members speak anymore. They appeared to become impatient. One or two left the room. Finally, the sound came back on. The doctor who asked the question replied that yes, oxybutynin was available. Dr. Das explained that oxybutynin was the drug of choice. It did have some side effects, but the advantage was that you could give very small doses and frequency or interval could be decided according to the patient's needs. Suddenly, everyone in the room at the IIM burst out laughing. For several seconds, they laughed heartily. Dr. Das wondered what was going on. I suggested the most likely cause: they just saw me in the picture and were somewhat surprised to see a white man, clearly not an Indian, appear on the screen. Maybe they made sense of where that Quebecois accent was coming from. Once things calmed down, Dr. Das asked whether there were any more questions. There was none. Dr. Das thanked the audience for their time before getting up and leaving the studio.

My involvement in translation tasks remained somewhat anecdotal. However, it pointed toward linguistic barriers that were not limited to CME sessions and were a continuous obstacle to communication in PAN. Just think of the dozens of engineers dispatched to cities, regions, and countries where they did not speak the language. The task of engineers was thus complicated by language barriers, as they sought to establish links with doctors, departments, and host institutions. In short, the decision to address the diverse linguistic landscape of the network's wide coverage area by using a lingua franca brought with it numerous challenges that impacted the use of services. Participants, in any case, were unanimous: language complicated the communication on the network.

In addition to language barriers, technical limitations also disturbed communication over the network. Although the video quality was generally considered acceptable, the high latency of the satellite connection caused delays in voice transmission, affecting the fluidity of conversations. A neurologist at CHNU Fann noted, "Communication is difficult over the network. We struggle to properly hear each other's voices. And then there is the accent. We need to make a huge effort to communicate."[26] Such comments were illustrated in many cases presented in this book, with doctors having to complete teleconsultations by chatting, which entailed exercising a great deal of patience. While the picture quality was generally considered acceptable, the difficulties were primarily with the audio. The sound was regularly cut off, and the latency made conversations difficult. The time lag between the moment a doctor spoke and the moment their colleague heard them was a source of confusion that was deplored as a loss of spontaneity. This technical limitation was directly related to the choice of satellite connectivity as well as to the spatial ordering of the network in a star topology—both of which exacerbated the latency. It was also possible to interrogate the relevance of videoconferencing, considering that a telephone conversation or an exchange of emails could sometimes have been more efficient. However, the actual impact of technical issues on the rate of utilization of the network should not be taken for granted. Most doctors remained relatively satisfied with the quality of communication. Even when technical problems were experienced as irritants, it was not easy to assess the extent of the relation between this dissatisfaction and any reluctance to use the network. All in all, technical communication issues may have been a contributing factor but not a decisive one.

Organization and Method

"It's a question of organization and method," suggested Dr. Diop at CHNU Fann when discussing the poor utilization of PAN. Many participants had strong opinions on the network's design, management, and daily operations. They attributed the project's low utilization to its design and especially to the weak organizational and spatial integration of the network within hospitals. PAN was designed to *first* connect sites and *then* integrate them into their host institution. It was not expected to emerge from local practices but to graft onto them. However, PAN did not blend easily within participating hospitals. The project was highly standardized, with the same medical expertise, equipment, schedules, and technical protocols expected to be used everywhere. The project's design aimed to be operational in any institutional setting. What I earlier referred to as its "portability kit" ensured the network's stability and autonomy regarding connectivity, power supply, and skilled labor. However, as discussed in chapter 3, this autonomy resulted in PAN being isolated from the sites where it was implemented.

In addition to spatial remoteness, PAN suffered from poor organizational integration. This was evident in the selection of personnel involved in its daily operations, starting with the on-site engineers. TCIL assigned engineers to all participating hospitals, with the expectation that they would promote the project and build relationships with local doctors. However, this seldom occurred. Engineers were selected based on their technical training and skills rather than their ability to raise local awareness about the project. Since most engineers were of Indian origin, they often knew very little about their assigned sites before arrival and had to adapt quickly. This modus operandi stemmed from PAN's turnkey approach, which aimed to standardize the training and work of engineers. An official at the African Union Commission explained, "Nobody could interfere with India on that front because they had decided to give the network on a turn-key basis."[27]

Many doctors practicing at CHNU Fann believed that issues such as the weak integration of the project, the selection of involved personnel, and the lack of strong relationships between doctors were ultimately the outcome of a lack of flexibility, which was embedded in the project from the design stage. "It is not flexible, not customized," a Senegalese neurologist remarked, explaining why he did not attend CME sessions provided by the project, even though he regularly used the network for teleconsultations. The CME program, which struggled to attract an audience, was frequently cited as an illustration of this inflexibility. One major issue was scheduling conflicts.[28] Doctors at CHNU Fann felt that the CME sessions were poorly timed since they were mostly broadcast in the morning when the doctors were busy visiting inpatients in their departments.[29] Scheduling conflicts also occasionally affected teleconsultations. Given the involvement of many hospitals, each with its own schedule, these conflicts were difficult to avoid. In essence, the project linked too many hospitals in too many countries, making it challenging to adapt to their specific routines, practices, and needs. Dr Diop explained, "Underutilization exists because there is no need-based approach, so they have to be large. These are choices that have been made and imposed. We were offered a package. We have never been asked what our needs were."[30]

The project was systematically caught in between highly centralized management on the one hand and the singularity of local conditions and institutional settings on the other.[31] As a result, links between the network and participating institutions remained too often tenuous and unstable. The project struggled to create durable relations, including relations that might flourish outside of the parameters of the network per se. Doctors very rarely met outside of the project's platform.[32] Local adaptations were also at times prevented or hindered by the rigidity of the network infrastructure. When managers at CHNU Fann mentioned an intention to expand the network to other hospitals in Senegal, they were notified that the architecture of the network did not allow for such a makeshift expansion. This lack of adaptability was primarily the consequence of PAN's hub-and-spoke model. As explained in chapter 3, *hub-and-spoke* refers to a network topology in which all devices are connected to a central hub. Hub-and-spoke also is a business model in which "spokes"—here, connected hospitals—are vertically integrated into a larger network while flows of data, goods, services, or information are managed by the hub. The hub-and-spoke model, however, did not allow for connections to be established directly between African hospitals. As a result, there was very little place for organic growth in PAN. To borrow the language of organizational studies, PAN did not allow for emergent organizational change—for change that arises from an unplanned, bottom-up process of transformation rather than from a predetermined model set by leadership.[33] The hub-and-spoke, along with the turnkey approach to project development, expressed underlying dreams of control and prediction.[34] But they also made PAN susceptible to the high levels of uncertainty inherent to the complex environments in which it evolved.

PAN produced new patterns of spatial organization among doctors, hospitals, and countries. Following a hub-and-spoke model, the network appeared to hover above African sites, which were integrated, and subordinated within higher-order connections. Fantasies of smooth integration and indeed of a unified and uniform South-South sphere of exchange disregarded the singularity of connected sites with their situated medical knowledge and practices.[35] Everything seemed as though the network preexisted, autonomous from the peoples, sites, and relations that effectively composed it. The next sections attend to this distancing and some of its consequences.

The Network and Its Other

"Whatever attendance is there, there is nothing wrong on the part of the network itself. It is there and it works great," insisted a former chairman of TCIL when asked to comment on the poor utilization of the Pan-African e-Network. While seemingly innocuous, this statement revealed much about the network's design. Put simply, the statement implied that PAN was merely a technical tool available for potential users. As a matter of fact, *that* network functioned relatively well. With few exceptions, the equipment had been delivered and installed, engineers were stationed, and data was circulating. However, the statement also highlighted the extent to which PAN's conception was premised on an ontological distinction between technical and nontechnical domains.[36]

This pattern was common in explanations for the low utilization of the Pan-African e-Network. As mentioned earlier, factors such as African doctors' reluctance to use it were viewed merely as obstacles to the project—minor setbacks or unfortunate mishaps. Anything that called into question the network's design and the vision of the future it carried was systematically dismissed as temporary or extraneous. This was most clearly expressed by TCIL's insistence that the primary reason for the network's low utilization was a lack of awareness. As it implied that the main obstacle was simply that people were unaware of or misunderstood the network, the focus on awareness validated the network in its original form. According to its designers and implementers, the essence of the project was beyond reproach: the tool was properly designed and only needed to be used correctly.

Literature about global health, including ethnographic research, tends to insist on the necessity to take "local contexts" into consideration in the design of specific interventions and projects. This includes literature about the rapid expansion of digital health in sub-Saharan Africa. Literature insists on the need for interventions to be home based or at least involving local actors from an early stage, cost effective, sensitive to social and economic determinants of health, and culturally and technologically adapted to the local conditions (Olu et al. 2019; van Stam 2022). Local communities should also identify the problems addressed by digital health technologies, and projects should be designed and implemented using a collaborative approach.[37] This was not the case for the Pan-African e-Network. As the network was implemented and utilization issues arose, local conditions of all sorts caught the attention of PAN's managers. But there was little they could do about it. TCIL was a technology company, and as its chairman had explained to me, as far as technology was concerned, PAN was doing fine. Things like language barriers, time zones, and the frustrations and resistance of local doctors were always imagined to be exterior to the network infrastructure itself. But most importantly, distancing and disengagement from local conditions was not an anomaly in PAN. Rather, it was deliberately inscribed in its design. As the saying goes, distance was not a bug; it was a feature.

As discussed in previous chapters, PAN depended upon movements of enclosure. These movements took many different forms. Enclosure was commercial: the hub-and-spoke model structured circulation over the network, thus borrowing from the expansion of telemedicine in India, which aimed at the vertical integration of hospitals. Enclosure was also infrastructural as it aimed to design lived environments, or milieus, suited for remote medicine. Hence the portability kit, designed to stabilize the practical conditions under which the network would operate and order the coexistence of beings and things in space.

PAN was premised on precisely this notion that it should be guarded from unforeseen conditions and events. The project exhibited an unrelenting quest for mastery, exemplified by the choice to adopt a turnkey approach for implementation. A turnkey, centralized, and standardized strategy was deemed the only viable solution for the project. It was expected to turn heterogeneous practices and processes into standardized and manageable activities and outcomes. One of the ways this was done was by maintaining a divide between technical and nontechnical domains—specifically, between PAN and the contexts in which it was being implemented, which were systematically made into the "other" of the network.[38]

The turnkey approach, and the implied division between what was and what was not the network, was integral to PAN. However, as I have suggested in chapter 2, in practice PAN did not preexist the people, relations, and things that composed it. It emerged out of material and practical relations. Its stability had to be enacted through constant labor and care. For some time already, social scientists and philosophers have examined how science and technology thus shape or, rather enact, their objects in practice.[39] Attempting to move beyond the dichotomy between being and representing—or between reality and our representational access to it—this body of work does not seek to formulate a theory of being or to claim access to reality as it is, as a reference to ontology could otherwise suggest. By contrast, it empirically investigates how relational, multiple, and more or less indeterminate practices are involved in world-making processes (Law and Lien 2013, 365). The aim is to describe and conceptualize the crystallization of specific objects and ontological formations, just like PAN, out of infinitely varied elements (Gad, Jensen, and Winthereik 2015, 83).

Importantly for this discussion, exploring how objects are enacted in practice implies a refusal to draw on context as an explanatory or descriptive tool.[40] The issue with PAN was not that context was not properly taken into consideration when designing the network. It was not that designers were ineffective in matching the technology to contexts in which it was implemented. The embeddedness and sheer materiality of the network cannot be reduced to a mere matter of accounting for given contexts. Similarly, the enclosure of PAN was not only an issue of distance vis-á-vis preexisting contexts. Rather, the issue was that context was conceived as a stable, static entity, as something surrounding the network—and, therefore, from which the network could and should be protected. In other words, the issue with the divide between technical and nontechnical domains was not only that it sustained the fantasy of a pure, non-context-specific technology, as it surely did. It was also that the project failed to *contextualize* itself, to give itself a context (Latour 1996). What did PAN effectively pass on to larger economic, medical, and social environments?

For engineers and managers working on PAN, the network was first a technological device, the equipment of which had to be maintained.[41] The dismissal of nontechnical processes and realities as anecdotal, however, came at a cost. It entailed a constant struggle to shield the project against possible contamination from the outside. Such habitations of distance have a long history in technopolitical interventions. One can, for instance, think of James C. Scott's magisterial critique of top-down social and technocratic planning and of a hegemonic planning mentality that excludes local knowledge. In *Seeing Like a State*, Scott explains how, to understand the failure of so many schemes aimed at improving the human condition, one has to contrast "high-modernist" views with critical perspectives that emphasize process, complexity, and open-endedness (Scott 1998, 6). Scott famously frames this contrast as a matter of vision and, most specifically, of legibility. He shows how certain technologies—of naming, accounting, classifying, and so on—make certain things and not others visible to the eye of the state. Here, *making visible* refers to making legible, commensurable, and accountable. The gaze of the state, Scott insists, is not able to properly handle complexity: achieving control depends on a simplified and reductionist view of the world.

Thinking like a state, suggests Bruno Latour, commenting Scott's thesis, is premised on the notion that calculation could *replace* politics. Ultimately, the heart of the matter boils down to a matter of political epistemology, of confusion between the world and its representation: "The many catastrophes reviewed by James Scott in his book, have all been caused by this confusion between the map and the territory—give me the map, and I will reshape the territory!" (Latour 2007b, 5). To inquire over a public problem, notes Latour, such state thinking—or seeing, for Scott—relies on a "view from above." This is a very specific way to account for a problem and make it legible. In contrast, addressing the problem in all of its intricacies entails experimental and carefully accountable procedures of inquiries aimed at describing, assembling, and composing: it requires politics. The issue with PAN, then, was not so much the role played by vested interests and political passions in imagining, designing, and implementing the network. Rather, the issue laid in the idea that PAN could neutralize the messiness of the sites that were not simply connected by the network but were actually composing it. Even as PAN dreamt of closure and control, it could work only by proliferating difference. This conviction that it was always possible and desirable to preserve the project against outside influences was thus central to the poor utilization of the Pan-African e-Network. To borrow another image from Latour, PAN was like a moralist: its hands were clean, but it did not have hands (Latour 1996, 127).

Too Big to Fail

"Being the President he had the power to do this. He had the imagination to do this. He's a scientist," explained a former scientist involved in telemedicine at the Indian Space Research Organisation (ISRO).[42] When I suggested that Dr. Kalam perhaps did not entirely conceive of the Pan-African e-Network on its own, the ISRO scientist insisted the vision of the network came out of the president's mind.

For most PAN actors, the story of President Kalam's original vision of the network often appeared to have quasi-mythological status. As the story went, Dr. Kalam first imagined the whole network, which was then implemented by scientists, engineers, and managers. "Dr. Kalam, he thinks big. It was his vision!" were the words of a former TCIL executive, already cited in the introduction of the book.

The story of Kalam's vision was indeed a story about scale and thinking big. The story described the origins of a colossal gift—India's largest single development project and one of the world's widest telemedicine networks. What seemed to be at stake in Kalam's vision was its power to make us imagine globality and speculate on a world to come. As examined in chapter 4, PAN was the object of great affective and imaginative investment. As a gift, PAN reconceptualized and reorganized spatial relations between countries and continents. PAN truly was a *scaling* project that relied on a significant work of imagination. Kalam's radiating charisma did not do the trick alone. Things like the footprint of the Rascom-QAF1R satellite, the promise of South-South cooperation, and the hub-and-spoke model were also drawn together in making it possible to imagine globality and how it might succeed (Tsing 2005, 57).

The scaling of PAN was at once speculative and practical, which translated into specific design choices, starting with the decision to expand the network fast and wide: TCIL would connect over forty hospitals within a few months. In talking with engineers and managers who were involved in laying out the network on either the Indian or the African side of it, it became evident that Kalam's vision did not materialize easily. The growth of the network was not organic or spontaneous, and it involved various kinds of labor from the beginning. During the two years following President Kalam's announcement, long hours were spent at the drawing table. There were debates and conflicting views of what form the network should take. A joint committee composed of members of ISRO, the Department of Telecommunications, and technology experts at Rashtrapati Bhavan (Office of the President) drafted an initial report. Prepared over a period of four months, the report was coordinated by the Ministry of External Affairs (MEA) of India. The project was then presented to a technical committee of the African Union and revised after discussions. Soon, TCIL, a government-owned engineering and consultancy company already active in Africa, was selected to implement the network. On October 27, 2005, a memorandum of understanding between India and the African Union was signed. On July 5, 2007, the project budget was approved by the government of India. The very next day, a pilot project connecting India with Ethiopia was inaugurated by Pranab Mukherjee, the minister of external affairs of India. As part of the pilot, the CARE hospital in Hyderabad was connected to the Black Lion Hospital in Addis Ababa and Nekempte Hospital in rural Ethiopia over the course of several months. The pilot faced many challenges, both technical and organizational. Connectivity was erratic, and participation was low. However, the issues experienced by the pilot did not dampen the spirits of the PAN implementers. The vision of President Kalam remained whole. Over the following months, TCIL started to implement the network infrastructure across the African continent. Satellite dishes were installed. Memoranda of understanding (MoU) were signed. As a result, more or less two years after the pilot had started its activities, the Pan-African e-Network was officially inaugurated on February 26, 2009. Soon enough, more than thirty countries over two continents were connected.

As an organizational form, however, the hub-and-spoke topology did not scale easily. Obstacles were plenty. The first major challenge was found in the circulation of things. Suppliers under contract to TCIL were in charge of shipping the project equipment to each country. Shipping was primarily by air and sea (as in the case of uninterruptible power systems). But the movement of equipment was not always smooth. On occasion, computer and medical equipment sent from India sat in airport hangars for months. Customs clearance procedures are not the same everywhere and could be very complex, much to the dismay of TCIL officials. As a result, storage fees could accumulate quickly and even result in equipment being tied up until the fees were paid. For example, when I visited the project's premises in Egypt, PAN's medical program had not yet begun as the equipment was awaiting customs clearance. It was explained to me that when donated equipment was imported, the procedure had to go through the prime minister's office, which could cause additional delays. On other occasions, countries held back on the exemption of customs duties for imported materials. In one case, former chairman and managing director Vimal Wakhlu explained, TCIL had to shell out its own money to get customs clearance (BT Bureau 2015).

The circulation of equipment was also not always straightforward within countries and hospitals. Once the equipment arrived at its destination, it was not necessarily used as intended. At CHNU Fann, there was a mobile X-ray machine on the floor that had never been taken out of its box: the hospital was already equipped with a better version of the machine, and it was being used for the project. On other occasions, equipment intended for the project was dispatched to other departments and used for different purposes. Whether locally or transnationally, the circulation of things was thus volatile, unpredictable, and contingent on a wide array of environmental factors that were not under TCIL's control. They did not travel along expected paths—namely, between a central location and several spokes leading out from that hub.

The mobility of the personnel was also an issue. As mentioned earlier, TCIL mostly employed Indian engineers. However, convincing engineers to move and work on the African sites of the network was apparently not easy. I was often reminded that in the popular imagination, living in Africa—or at least in some countries—was associated with all kinds of hardships and dangers. As mentioned earlier, when discussing the risks associated with PAN, an officer at the Ministry of External Affairs suggested that Indian engineers working on the project were concerned that they may not come back alive. Stereotypes, prejudice, and ill representation of the African continent thus complicated the recruitment of Indian engineers.

The scaling of PAN also came with logistics challenges. Extending the network implied dealing with many service and technology providers as well as with government agencies. Abiding by government rules often involved tedious and complex procedures. In practical terms, bilateral agreements (MoUs) had to be signed with every country. Since joining the project was not mandatory, TCIL could not easily anticipate how many and which countries would eventually be joining the network and when they would do so. This, in turn, complicated procurement. How, a TCIL official complained to me, could the company estimate the network's future requirements for materials, goods, and services? How could it manage advanced purchase orders and get the best quotes from manufacturers without knowing how many sites would be connected? These logistic challenges made visible the state of constant improvisation that PAN managers were in to expand and stabilize the network.

In business and technology literature, hub-and-spoke topologies have a reputation of easy scalability. Additional devices can be easily added to the network by connecting them to the hub, making it simple to expand the network without any significant changes to the existing infrastructure. Since all devices connect to the hub, it can be upgraded to have more ports and connect more sites without having to change the devices on the network. The experience of PAN complicates such claims. The struggle to expand PAN reminds us that scales are not ontological givens: they are actively produced. Scales are processes before they are products (Carr and Lempert 2016). The writings of Anna Tsing on logics of scale are particularly instructive in that regard. Scalability, Tsing explains, is "the ability of a project to change scales smoothly without any change in project frames" (2015, 38). Scale requires that project elements be "oblivious to the indeterminacies of encounter; that's how they allow smooth expansion" (38). Making projects scalable thus demands a lot of work. Scales must be brought into being through all sorts of commitments and practices.[43] For Tsing, scaling is not a neutral process. It comes with significant social and ecological consequences. Scaling often involves the creation of new hierarchies, which can lead to the marginalization of certain groups and the concentration of power in the hands of a few. Hence, a theory of nonscalability should start by attending to the work it takes to scale projects but also to the messes it makes. In other words, to learn about the big, universalizing forces at work in a project like PAN, "we have to pay attention to what happens when they meet and collide with particular situations" (Wark 2016).

As I have tried to show in different ways throughout this book, the peoples and places connected via PAN often had little in common. PAN could scale only by linking dissimilar sites. This included hospitals with varying health landscapes, languages, modes of operation, and technology. It also included distinctive border politics, bureaucracies, national interests, local infrastructure, and workforces. Under these conditions, the hub-and-spoke topology ensured close control over the network's expansion as well as over data flows. It also provided a model for economic growth, with local hospitals being vertically integrated within a transnational infrastructure of expertise and care. Life in PAN was thus governed and supported through a material form that conditioned interactions at a distance. It simultaneously intensified and ordered the circulation of knowledge between participating hospitals. As a result, connections between patients, doctors, and hospitals were heavily patterned, and some actors were confined to limited roles.

PAN's scaling challenges, as well as its low utilization, can be read as a (partially) failed attempt to integrate a continent *from above and beyond*. Low utilization also reveals a certain arrogance, or conceit, in the notion that certain things can be built or operated anywhere, "regardless of the specificities of setting or the practicality of use" (Simone 2018). But it also raises a much more complicated question: What is the proper type of distanciation, which ensures a certain autonomy for a project while allowing connections to be established and relations to thrive? This is not an easy issue to settle. How is it possible, if at all, for a project like PAN to maintain its consistency while keeping open the possibility of other futures? How could PAN have scaled from the ground up? Remember the "single story" presented by Nolwazi Mkhwanazi earlier in this chapter: social science literature overwhelmingly focuses on the *unpredictability* of biomedical technologies and interventions implemented in sub-Saharan Africa. In contrast, PAN tells a story about how the specificity of peoples and things coexists with the wildest, most enduring dreams of expansion and universality.

Making Distance

Some dreams, write Wensel Geissler and Noémi Tousignant, "actively produce failures and contradictions that they are unable to effectively recognize or address" (Geissler and Tousignant 2020, 5). Dreams can drive an endless chase for a destination that can't ever be reached. PAN was the product of big dreams of expansion and integration, totality and verticality. As a speculative project, PAN sought to make the world in the image of such dreams.

Or, rather, in the image of a vision—Kalam's vision. As I have tried to show throughout this chapter, these dreams and visions haunted the design and deployment of PAN at every stage. PAN was designed to scale as a homogeneous, universalizing project. At the level of infrastructure and organization, it sought to establish uniformity in order to function well. It aspired to a perfect form imposed upon an environment with a promise to integrate a vast and rich terrain of experience into a cohesive, objective world. Making distance was the price to pay to keep the dream alive. PAN's movements of enclosure were thus not an anomaly or a failure.[44] As a scaling project, PAN was actively disengaged from the specificity of the hospitals it connected. This was done by design: PAN *demanded* such a habitation of distance. Different discourses, techniques, and imaginations contributed to performing distance. These included the hub-and-spoke topology, the satellite imagination, an emancipatory conception of digital technology, and market expansion projects using telemedicine, among other things.

I would like to conclude this chapter by emphasizing how distancing in PAN was not only infrastructural and spatial—it was also normative and political. Over the many conversations we have had about the network, PAN implementors have constantly insisted on the apparently poor state of tertiary medicine in Africa. There was a consensus that whether complemented by medical tourism or not, telemedicine could help build access. The vertical integration of African hospitals within a transnational network of care and expertise was seen as a solution for a situation of lack. PAN, again, was a gift that would contribute to expanding the reach of medical expertise, and of tertiary care in particular. However, the project concealed processes of differentiation and hierarchization inherent to global biomedicine. It also rendered local populations remote. PAN built connected enclaves of medical expertise, contributing to the fragmentation and uneven distribution of health care across the African continent. It produced an "imagined global community of remote medical professionals" (Cartwright 2000, 367) in need of foreign expertise and of being "brought up" into the network society. Access to the network was conceived as a condition to participating in global biomedicine. As is often the case with digital media, it was assumed to determine whether one is an "agent of history or a silent passenger, and thus, whether one is living in the present or the past" (Hirschkind, de Abreu, and Caduff 2017, S4). PAN was accompanied by aspirations to a universal that offered the chance "to participate in the global stream of humanity" (Tsing 2005, 6). Such a gift could hardly be turned down. In any case, it should not be. Recalcitrance to use the network was thus swiftly interpreted as resistance to change if not as a kind of ignorance. PAN presented African countries with a linear trajectory toward a future that India already inhabited, or at least Indian hospitals and technoscience.[45] In this teleological conception of development, African nations could only play catch-up from within the Global South.[46] They were othered as students while India produced a self-referential distinction as a model. Scales, after all, are ways of seeing and standing in the world (Carr and Lempert 2016, 10). Ethnographic attention to the experience on the network, including its low utilization, undoes any notion of a monolithic South. Rather, it hints at a multitude of divides and inequalities and indeed at the distribution of power from within the Global South. PAN, in other words, involved asymmetric power relations and installed distance between modelers and the people and sites (Viveiros de Castro 2019, S300).

At times, PAN was seen as a promising substitute for postcolonial trajectories of care whose approaches are considered dated, paternalistic, and opportunistic. At the very least, South-South cooperation projects such as PAN diversify Africa's economic partnerships, granting the continent new negotiating power. They provincialize Eurocentric spheres of development and global health in which the South is ever considered peripheral. Even as they genuinely welcomed the prospect of cooperation with Indian rather than Chinese or Western partners, it would be a mistake to confuse African actors with passive recipients of projects implemented from above.[47] Because of distance, PAN was not attentive to interruptions and deviations that could not be easily communicated or put into words. For example, it neglected the possibility that poor utilization may have expressed a passive form of resistance in which people simply did not use or engage with the project, rather than actively protesting or opposing it. The reluctance of African doctors to use the network, which some blamed on their professional ego, could at least partially be understood as noncompliance or noncooperation. There might have been deliberate avoidance or refusal to participate in a network that, after all, was suspected of producing new patterns of dependence on foreign expertise and technology. The same could be said of equipment blocked at customs or redistributed within hospitals, of engineers passing time, or of passivity promoting the network. Resistance to projects like PAN does not always speak its name.[48]

Framed in terms of visibility, it is possible that PAN's struggles with detecting the singularity of its terrain were also the result of an opacity that was, to some degree, *cultivated*. By opacity, I do not mean some sort of incommensurable ontological quality. Rather, opacity refers to a strategic withdrawal or refusal to participate. The writings of Martinican philosopher and poet Édouard Glissant come to mind. In *The Politics of Relations*, Glissant famously made an argument for the right to opacity. Opacity, he insisted, is "not enclosure within an impenetrable autarchy but subsistence within an irreducible singularity" (Glissant 1997, 190).[49] For Glissant, opacity disrupts the gaze and management of Western thought.[50] Against dreams of total integration and transparency, often carried by communication technologies such as the satellite, to remain opaque is to refuse to be included in universal models and categories. Transparency, for Glissant, operates a reduction. And it is very much central to the work of scale that, again, shall be understood not only in spatial but also in normative terms: not only as a measure of size but also as a *model* for futures to come. Opacity, then, may upset the hierarchy of an imposed ideal scale: "But perhaps we need to bring an end to the very notion of a scale. Displace all reduction" (190).

There is no reason to believe that nonusers or infrequent users of PAN opposed telemedicine per se.[51] Rather, they refused to engage with telemedicine under the terms of *that* network. When doctors and managers in Africa mentioned that PAN was not tailored for them, they deplored the impossibility of engaging the network in terms and scales that were their own—for example, imagining it otherwise, tinkering with it from the inside out. They refused to be peripheral nodes in a totalizing cartography of the world. They were not eager to participate in an either/or, take-it-or-leave-it approach and rejected the cynical position of the user. In other words, African (non)participants in PAN were unsatisfied with being passive recipients of foreign expertise and technology. They wanted to innovate, transform, and expand the network in new ways. PAN's model, however, which was at once an economic model and a topological form, largely undermined such possibility for a truly creative, open-ended engagement with the network. As artifacts of the project, for example, the enclosures produced by PAN were not fragments from which new relations could easily emerge and new medical worlds could be recomposed.

At stake here is the interplay of the singular and the universal. "True *care for the universal*," writes Senegalese philosopher Souleymane Bachir Diagne, "means *attention to the particular*" (Diagne 2013, 17). It is at the Bandung Conference, Diagne reminds us, that the notion of a new and genuine universal to be crafted emerged. At Bandung, the notion of the universal was de-Westernized, and Africa and Asia in particular affirmed their role in the writing of its history. Europe became an object and no longer the center of discourse—a provincializing gesture that augured the erosion of the colonial distance between center and periphery (Diagne 2017). Inspired by the works of Glissant but also of Léopold Sédar Senghor, Aimé Césaire, and Maurice Merleau-Ponty, Diagne proposes a notion of the universal crafted out of immanent relation.[52] The universal is always contingent on the incompleteness of translation. It is never fully present to itself.

PAN presented the world with convincing universals: biomedicine, network science, and, above all, Kalam's messianic vision of technology as a driver of economic growth and human development. However, these universals were over-hanging and dropped from above—from outer space, just like signals of the satel-lite. The network form was normative and political in the sense that it imposed order and reorganized spatial relations between continents. PAN respatialized an otherwise empty analytical category—the South—in relation to India, thus giving form to the nation as a real and imagined entity. In doing so, it also natu-ralized the boundaries of the African continent as a single domain of interven-tion. In quite a twist of history, PAN asserted new relations between center and periphery.[53]

Thus detailing the spatial form of global flows forces us to approach the intri-cate relations between movements of closure and the ever-elusive difference that is constitutive of network infrastructure. Years of ethnographic inquiries into medicine, science, and technology have revealed the extent to which territories can be opaque and recalcitrant: they exceed maps. Even enclosed territorialities may be rough, leaky, or vibrant with indeterminacy. We know, in other words, that abstraction into a traveling, universal form—here, the network form—is never total. It always leaves a remainder that won't be contained. And yet rec-ognizing this difference between map and territory is hardly sufficient to miti-gate the entrancing power of the network form. By representing the world, maps intervene in the world. Many participants in the Pan-African e-Network, after all, *believed* in the power of the network and acted accordingly. It is not satisfying to proclaim, once again, that the map is not the territory. Perhaps the map is just not the territory *yet*.

Epilogue

Wherever we look, the drive is toward enclosure.

—Achille Mbembe (2018)

"Today this project exists in many African countries and before its end in 2014, we believe African countries will be able to sustain it for the next generation," announced Mr. Vimal Wahklu at the launch of the PAN site in South Sudan, in the fall of 2012 (Joseph 2012). The statement by the new TCIL chairman summarized what was then the official plan for the future of PAN. According to the plan, TCIL and the government of India would implement and operate the network free of charge but for a limited time only. The Indian Ministry of External Affairs was to fund the network for a period of five years, from February 2009 to 2014, after which TCIL would hand over its control. In due time, PAN was expected to be operated in and from Africa. Specifically, the African Union Commission (AUC) would take over the network and turn it into a commercial enterprise.

The most likely scenario entailed handing over control of the network's operations to a commercial entity, the creation of which the AUC would oversee. It was never the AUC's mission to operate the network, even after Indian funding ran out: the organization planned to transfer ownership to an entity that would manage the network, develop its services further, and perhaps make a profit out of it. While the exact form that was to be taken by such a commercial entity was never fully determined, it seemed certain that Indian hospitals would remain involved as providers of medical care and expertise. A manager at Narayana Hrudayalaya Health City in Bangalore thus summarized the vision that many Indian stakeholders had of PAN's future: "Sooner or later, the African Union will take over the project and manage it themselves. And we could be their healthcare providers from here."[1] However, as was explained to me by an official at the AUC, PAN first had to become indispensable within the African health care landscape. African health care providers had to become "addicted first" to the services provided. Only then would PAN become sustainable and, hopefully, profitable. PAN was expected to become private but also to transform itself. In discussions I had with African actors of PAN, many evoked a decentralization of the network's operations. PAN would have to become more flexible and spread more easily. Some African participants insisted that they, and they only, could eventually extend the network to rural or remote regions. These futures, however, still have to materialize. In 2014, the government of India agreed to extend the funding of the project for three more years, following an official request formulated by the African Union. This new wave of funding covered operations for three more years.[2] But the question of how to turn the network into a profitable investment remained without a response. In July 2017, PAN officially ceased activities.

On September 10, 2018, the Ministry of External Affairs (MEA) of India, along with TCIL, signed the agreement for the implementation of the e-VidyaBharti and e-AarogyaBharti Network Project. Taking place in New Delhi, the signing ceremony was attended by M. J. Akbar, minister of external affairs of India, as well as by the African diplomatic corps, senior officials from the Department of Telecommunication, and representatives from Indian educational and health care institutions. e-VidyaBharti (Sanskrit for "Indian tele-education") and e-Aarogya-Bharti (Sanskrit for "Indian telemedicine") are expected to replace the Pan-African e-Network. Although this revamped version of the network (referred to by the acronym e-VBAB) was officially launched in October 2019, it was apparently still being rolled out at the moment of writing. What is presented as the "second phase" or a "technological extension" of the Pan-African e-Network similarly offers continuing medical education and medical teleconsultations—although more importance seems to be given to the tele-education component of the network, which offers higher-education programs. TCIL is still in charge of the network's operations that now depend on a different network infrastructure, revolving around web-based portals instead of peer-to-peer satellite connectivity. Engineers should no longer be dispatched to connected hospitals (Banik, Venkatachalam, and Modi 2023, 20). However, the most important change is perhaps to be found elsewhere—namely, in the affective life of the project, as it speculates on the conditions under which India and Africa will weave the paths that connect both regions in the future.

~~~

PAN was borne out of a historical moment in which South-South cooperation, corporate medicine, and the promise of digital technology met as entangled manifestations of global capital in the early twenty-first century. Retrospectively, however, it appears to have been a presage of important changes to come. Between the end of PAN in 2017 and the current implementation of e-VBAB, the world has experienced a global pandemic during which some of the conceptual and practical issues raised by PAN were brought up with unprecedented urgency.

First, the COVID-19 pandemic accelerated the expansion of digital medicine while breathing new life into its past promises. Inspired by capitalist fantasies of flow and connectivity that have naturalized the notion that goods, services, and information should be able to move without barriers, digital medicine promises new spatial configurations of care and expertise. It aims to short-circuit the lack of health care infrastructure to reach the remotest people and places. In a context where restricting physical contact was a key element of the pandemic response, digital medicine also promised hygienic, secure medical care. Dreams of digital health—now often called *tele-health* rather than *telemedicine*—are also alive and well in India. In fact, as telemedicine pioneer Dr. K. Gapanathy recently explained to me, the pandemic came as a huge opportunity for digital health in India, as it has spurred exponential growth. In India, he described, "digital health is not the future—it is the present. . . . We are no longer aiming to achieve world class—we are aiming to make the rest of the world want to achieve India class!! We do not follow advanced countries. We do not piggy back. We do not even leap frog— after all how far can a frog leap!!"[3] Without dismissing them altogether, ethnographic inquiries into PAN complicate such promises as they reveal conflicted, contradictory spaces and histories. By showing how connectivity can craft new medical enclosures, PAN is warning us against the temptation to fetishize digital health and its global flows of data, knowledge, and technology.

What is also particularly thought-provoking in Dr. Ganapathy's statement is the way it posits India as teacher or guide to follow in the making of digital health worldwide. This is a second line of inquiry that PAN precociously raised but that the COVID-19 pandemic made into an urgent and public object of debate. The COVID-19 pandemic contributed to emphasizing discourses, interests, and practices that diverge from those that are prevalent in Western-centric global health spheres. The pandemic has underlined the growing impact of rising powers such as India and China on the geopolitics of global health. Chinese health officials traveled west to support medical teams. India's role as the "pharmacy of the world" and as a provider of medical expertise also was on full display. As this book suggested, PAN challenged common assumptions about the circulation of technology and medicine along North-South geopolitical lines. It defied the simplistic notion that mimics the geopolitical categorizations that colonialism was built upon and according to which the Global South is an amorphous recipient of aid, health care, and technology. As a gift, PAN opened up future possibilities. As such, it was generally received with a certain degree of optimism by African participants. However, as discussed throughout this book, the network also embedded new geographies of power with asymmetries and historical legacies of their own. It is possible to think of PAN as a key component of India's growing global health diplomacy efforts. With the COVID-19 pandemic, India's health diplomacy shifted into high gear as it sought to influence the global health environment through various efforts (Chattu et al. 2023). For example, India and South Africa proposed a temporary waiver of intellectual property rights to the World Trade Organization (WTO) to ensure the timely affordability and accessibility of COVID-19 vaccines (Singh et al. 2023). Prime Minister Modi also energetically praised India's contribution to the global pandemic response as an illustration of vasudhaiva kutumbakam.[4]

Besides the pandemic, however, the past decade has witnessed many instances that brought critical attention to the global racial imaginaries that shape South-South cooperation, Indo-Africa encounters in particular. The legacy of the (post)colonial partnership between Africa and India has been the object of heated debate and new lines of resistance. Statues of Mohandas Gandhi were contested, removed, or vandalized in Africa amid a wider questioning of his legacy on the continent and his views on race in particular.[5] Then, multiple incidents of discrimination and violence faced by African students in India have also drawn attention to the rise of Afrophobia in the country. As was suggested by Jideofor Adibe (2017), these xenophobic attacks and the apparent failure of Indian authorities to forcefully condemn them could affect Afro-India relations. This includes the medical tourism industry, with media coverage of the attacks persuading African patients to move to other low-cost destinations. Most importantly, Afrophobia undercuts India's efforts to craft the imagination of a unique model of cooperation with Africa based on past experiences and shared solidarity and emphatically distinct from China's approach.

Simultaneously, the past decade has witnessed the rise to power of Hindu nationalists in India.[6] As I have suggested in this book, although the network was driven by a logic of market expansion, PAN materialized an affective investment in the future of the nation.

PAN was arguably President Kalam's project: it was a medium for the nation to perform itself as an aspirant ruler in a new world order. However, e-VBAB appears to gesture to a shift from Indian toward Hindu nationalism. In the words of Dr. S. Jaishankar, minister of external affairs of the government of India since 2019, beyond cooperation itself, e-VBAB underlines India's progressive emergence on the global stage (Jaishankar 2020). However, this new rendering of the network gives an overtly ethnonationalist turn to India's aesthetic of arrival on the world stage. It resonates with Prime Minister Modi's project to usher India into a new era of expansion driven by a mix of realpolitik and Hindu nationalist ambition. This is illustrated by the new Sanskrit appellation and the inclusion of Bharat (the name of India in Hindu antiquity) in the project's name.[7]

At home, too, India has been increasingly recast as a Hindu majoritarian nation where minorities, especially Muslims, are second-class citizens—a dynamic of exclusion that has been facilitated and legitimized by digital technology. On the occasion of his passing in July 2015, Dr. Kalam was himself referred to as a great nationalist "despite being a Muslim" by the minister of culture under the Modi government in power. The shameful statement, for which he was not criticized within the party, captures the normalization of anti-Muslim rhetoric within Indian politics and the fragility of the exceptional status awarded to Kalam as a "good Muslim." Such a statement appears as one more indication that e-VBAB is no longer Kalam's project. In PAN, the logic of global capital and the celebration of civilizational difference reinforced each other. But civilizational difference was not laid out in the ethnic terms that compose the kind of Hindu nationalism found under the leadership of Narendra Modi. Under Modi, notions such as South-South solidarity and decolonization are increasingly mobilized as an appendage to Brahmanic or Hindu supremacy. So is vasudhaiva kutumbakam, which occupies a prominent position in Modi's brand of Hindu nationalism.[8] Gift giving, then, is "increasingly viewed in relation to Indic frames of reference" (Banik and Mawdsley 2023, 544), and the idea that "India is a teacher of the world ('Vishwaguru')" (546) is more than ever mobilized, which may also cultivate a sense of inequality between partners of South-South cooperation, and especially between giver and recipient. In other words, African-Indian differences and hierarchies are increasingly used as "evidence of Indian universalism and justification for paternalism toward Africa" (Shankar 2021, 19). The way Africa has historically shaped and challenged India—and continues to do so—is not acknowledged, as the South serves as the ahistorical, enchanted space, through which the power of the nation is cultivated, again and again.

~~~

When I last visited CHNU Fann, Barrirou Ngom was sitting quietly at a desk, a few doors away from where the studios of the Pan-African e-Network used to be. After having obtained his PhD in France, Ngom had moved back to Senegal two years earlier. He had then accepted a position that would put him in charge of the technical components of telemedicine at CHNU Fann. Soon, however, telemedicine at Fann had almost ground to a halt. In November 2021, Ngom was working alone in his office. The whole floor was almost vacant. The Pan-African e-Network had been shut down for a few years already. Very little had moved in the large room in which its studios were once hosted. Some chairs and desks were scattered all over the place. The server room was still crowded with hardware, including servers, and UPS systems. Some other materials had been mobilized for other telemedicine activities at CHNU Fann. The satellite antenna was still sitting on the top of the building but was not used anymore: the hospital now had a decent landline Internet connection.

While some of the material infrastructure of the Pan-African e-Network was waiting to be reassembled into a new, enigmatic network, care work at Fann was being extended via other historical, well-trodden paths. For example, the Centre Cardio-pédiatrique Cuomo was launched at CHNU Fann in January 2017. The result of a 7 million euros investment by a private donor, Elena Cuomo, and under the leadership of La Chaîne de l'Espoir (the charity that had transferred nine-year-old Mamadou to the United Kingdom, among others, a few years before), the Centre Cardio-pédiatrique Cuomo became the first pediatric cardiology center in West Africa. Since 2017, it trains health care teams so that they can operate patients locally. Apparently hundreds of surgeries have since been performed on young patients, coming from all over West Africa. Thanks to the Centre Cardio-pédiatrique Cuomo, CHNU Fann is now more than ever a regional hub for hospital care.

A few months prior to my own visit, in 2021, officials from the African Union (AU) also came to tour the premises. They wanted to see what was left of PAN, and how some of it could be salvaged for e-AarogyaBharti. Barrirou Ngom knew very little about this new, revamped version of the network. The AU officials, he mentioned, had specified that CHNU Fann was one of the sites that had been best maintained since PAN was terminated. That was something to be proud of. After all, he was the one who had been left dealing with the debris of the network. Whenever the new project came, Barrirou Ngom would be ready.

Notes

INTRODUCTION

1. The name has been changed to assure confidentiality. Throughout the book I only name interlocutors who are public figures or who have clearly expressed the preference to have their name published.

2. The Pan-African e-Network also ran an extensive tele-education program in which African students enrolled in Indian universities. This book is concerned only with the telemedicine component of the network, including its Continuing Medical Education program, which was considered part of telemedicine. Although tele-education and tele-medicine were funded by the Ministry of External Affairs as parts of PAN and administered by TCIL, they connected different sites and offered very different services. I did not conduct any extensive fieldwork on tele-education sites. My analysis of PAN, therefore, is restricted to its telemedicine program. For a recent review of the project's tele-education program, see Banik, Venkatachalam, and Modi 2023.

3. Actual costs are hard to verify. In the course of this research, I have come across or heard about a whole range of estimations. US$200 million is the official figure published by the African Union in the *First Progress Report of the Chairperson of the Commission on the Pan-African E-Network on Tele-Education and Tele-Medicine*. The report is available here: https://au.int/sites/default/files/documents/34076-doc-auc.report.panafrican.e-net work.prc_.29.03.pdf.

4. This book speaks about PAN in the past tense, given that this new version of the network has been launched and advertised precisely as this: a new version. The technical infrastructure of this revamped network has been redesigned. The network was also given a new Sanskrit designation: e-VidyaBharti and e-ArogyaBharti, which may be respectively translated as e-Knowledge India and e-Health India. The network, one is tempted to suggest, has found its Hindu form. I examine these changes, and the kinds of futures they suggest, in the epilogue.

5. The Pan-African e-Network Project was indeed a project in the sense defined by Anna Tsing: "I use the term *projects* to mean organized packages of ideas and practices that assume an at least tentative stability through their social enactment, whether as custom, convention, trend, clubbish or professional training, institutional mandate, or government policy. A project is an institutionalized discourse with social and material effects" (Tsing 2001, 4).

6. Whether it be by policymakers, practitioners, or marketers, historian Jeremy Greene suggests, electronic media in medicine have constantly been a site for cultural and financial speculation. Greene writes, "When a new medium of clinical care is initially conceived and promoted to the medical profession and the lay public, it is suspended in a froth of enthusiasm between the interests of speculative research, speculative fiction, and speculative capital. . . . Each new electronic medium was initially borne aloft on a wave of speculation, a sea of stories predicting how it would revolutionize medical knowledge and clinical practice" (Greene 2022, 6).

7. Teleconsultations were not the only medical service offered by the Pan-African e-Network. As suggested in the description that opened this introduction, the network also delivered a comprehensive continuing medical education program. Broadcast live in participating hospitals, CME sessions consisted of daily sessions of live medical training.

Every Indian hospital offered six sessions per month covering a broad range of topics and specialties. As many as seventy-two sessions were thus broadcast every month in participant hospitals.

8. I borrowed this expression from Barry Saunders (2008).

9. Interview with the author, Dakar. Note that throughout the book, the dates of interviews are not included in order to help protect the anonymity of the interviewees.

10. Over the past decade or so, social studies of digital health have contributed to debunking such claims. Studies have insisted on the enduring relevance of place in digital health and critically examined the framing of digital medicine in terms of flow, transmission, and mobility (Oudshoorn 2012; Mort, Finch, and May 2009). They have insisted on the difficulty in predicting the way technologies and users would behave and emphasized the fluidity and relationality inherent to concrete health care situations and practices (Moser and Law 2006; Jensen 2010). Others have challenged widespread discourses that tend to associate telemedicine with coldness, rationality, and instrumentality, in contrast with the assumed proximity and warmth of human care (Pols and Moser 2009). It should be noted, however, that with few exceptions, social studies of telemedicine and digital health have been focusing overwhelmingly on Western contexts, with little attention being paid to the Global South. For exceptions, see Al Dahdah 2017, 2019; Duclos 2015, 2017; Miscione 2007; Neumark and Prince 2021; and Sawadogo et al. 2021.

11. Over the past decades, a range of otherwise disparate theorists—at times assembled under categories such as *actor-network theory*, *posthumanism*, or *new materialisms*—have insisted on how humans and tools continually modify each other and how technicity is from the onset constitutive of how humans come into being with the world. The arguments developed in this book have, in one way or another, been inspired by readings of scholars that include Madeleine Akrich, Karen Barad, Donna Haraway, Brian Larkin, Bruno Latour, Gilbert Simondon, Peter Sloterdijk, and Bernard Stiegler.

12. This is best illustrated by Susan Leigh Star's important work on the ethnography of infrastructure. For seminal papers, see Star and Ruhleder 1996; Star 1999; and Bowker and Star 1999.

13. Throughout the book, the names of all patients have been changed to ensure confidentiality.

14. For important ethnographic studies of improvisation in hospital care, see Livingston 2012 and Street 2014.

15. In spite of such a centralized approach, it should be noted that African partners also played a role, even though less visible, in setting up PAN. The African Union Commission assisted in laying out the network while host countries facilitated (or not) the circulation of equipment, identified the sites to be connected, and provided physical infrastructure within those sites.

16. UPS stands for "uninterruptible power supply." It is a power system that provides backup electrical power. PAN designers considered that a UPS was necessary to support the network in case of unstable power supply in a participating hospital.

17. For a discussion of the dialectics of speed and inertia in the context of global capital and what it might mean for social sciences, see Duclos, Sánchez Criado, and Nguyen 2017.

18. I also borrow the figure of the archipelago from P. Wenzel Geissler (2014), who writes about the archipelago of public health and science in African contexts.

19. This applies to global health, with its traditional emphasis on transnational mobilities which tends to conceal the importance of place, as well as new claims for nationhood and territory. See Anderson 2014. Chapter 5 examines how this played out in PAN.

20. *Economic* because it was inextricably linked to the establishment of a new economic order, itself based on strong a nation-building program. *Political* given that freedom and

equality could acquire significance only through the self-determination of member states. As noted by Partha Chatterjee, while liberty and equality were "key normative concepts animating the struggles of anticolonial nationalism," they were rights "claimed collectively by peoples" (Chatterjee 2017, 86). And finally, *technoscientific* given that science and technology formed the backbone of Nehru's efforts to redress a series of basic social problems both in India and abroad. More on this in chapter 1.

21. It should be noted, however, that India did deliver a telemedicine network to South Asian countries via the launch of the SAARC Telemedicine Network. SAARC stands for the South Asian Association for Regional Cooperation and comprises India, Bangladesh, Bhutan, Nepal, Pakistan, Sri Lanka, Afghanistan, and Maldives. Funded by the Indian Ministry of External Affairs and implemented by TCIL, the SAARC Telemedicine Network provides teleconsultation services to hospitals in Bhutan (Thimphu), Nepal (Kathmandu), and Afghanistan (Kabul). Two public Indian hospitals, SGPGIMS (Lucknow) and PGIMER (Chandigarh), are connected to the network. The SAARC Telemedicine Network is much smaller in scale than PAN and does not come with the same commercial ambitions.

22. For updated data, see https://wits.worldbank.org/CountryProfile/en/Country/SSF/StartYear/2013/EndYear/2017/TradeFlow/Import/Indicator/MPRT-TRD-VL/Partner/IND/Product/All-Groups.

23. See Banerjee 2017; Meier zu Biesen 2018; and Peterson 2014 for ethnographic accounts of pharmaceutical exchanges between India and Africa.

24. Interview with the author, New Delhi.

25. Interview with the author, Addis Ababa.

26. For a discussion of the aesthetics of India's arrival on the global stage, see Kaur and Blom Hansen 2016.

27. For a fine analysis of the symbolic power of foreign aid as gift, see Ilan Kapoor 2008. Kapoor argues that "aid giving is strongly allied with the production of the nation, where the construction of a positive, single national identity is paramount, and hence where the nation's aid as 'gift' trumps its grift" (Kapoor 2008, 78). While Kapoor focuses on Western foreign aid, which is constructed as unreciprocated, Mawdsley (2012) argues that by contrast, South-South cooperation insists on the "positive moral valence of reciprocity," thus challenging the dominant aid paradigm. Chapter 1 shows how PAN stands as a shining example of such moral claims. Chapter 4 discusses how theories of gift exchange can illuminate PAN's relationship to time as a project.

28. Although it was involved at the early stages of its design, ISRO did not play a key role in the implementation of PAN. More on this later.

29. See http://www.isro.gov.in.

30. As was noted in the Eleventh Five Year Plan (2007–12) published by the Planning Commission of India, the growth of the private sector in health care took place in the context of a failing public sector, and it was also directly encouraged by various public policies: "We have a flourishing private sector, primarily because of a failing in the public sector" (Planning Commission 2008, 67). On the privatization of the hospital sector, see also Lefebvre 2010 and Vaguet 2009. I examine this question in much more detail in chapter 1.

31. For an ethnography of the making of "entrepreneurial citizens" in India, see Irani 2019.

32. Hirschkind, de Abreu, and Caduff (2017, S4) make a similar argument: "Political and economic divides are increasingly recast as digital divides, while extending digital infrastructure around the globe is increasingly seen as a solution to diminish global inequalities."

33. As was noted by William Mazzarella (2010), perhaps nowhere was the promise that the internet was the "appropriate technology" for poverty reduction and development more intensely cultivated than in India. For an eminent example of such a narrative, see Nilekani 2009.

34. In the words of Kalam, an inspirational dreamer of revived national greatness: "Ancient India was a knowledge society and a leader in many intellectual pursuits, particularly in the fields of mathematics, medicine and astronomy. A renaissance is imperative for us to once again become a knowledge superpower rather than simply providing cheap labor in areas of high technology" (Kalam 2003, 38). India, in the most hopeful visions of the future, appears as the motherland of the digital. The invention of the zero, the age-old wrestling with the abstract concepts of the Upanishads, or a long-standing contempt for manual labor would stand as so much evidence of such a future ascent. In *India Unbound, Times of India* columnist Gurcharan Das encapsulates the argument: "We have wrestled with the abstract concepts of the Upanishads for three thousand years. We invented the zero. Just as spiritual space is invisible, so is cyberspace. Hence, our core competence is invisible. In information technology we may have finally found the engine that can drive India's takeoff and transform our country" (Das 2002, xvii). For critical discussion of the entanglement of Hindu nationalism with science and technology, see Chopra 2008; Prasad 2018; and Subramaniam 2019.

35. Kaur writes, "Capital appears as a curative force that can even redeem the nation's lost glory via economic growth. It is not just the infusion of capital that is critical in the making of the brand new nation; equally critical is the recognition of the nation's growth story by global capital. Thus, twentieth-century *nation building* is increasingly being replaced by twenty-first-century *nation branding*" (Kaur 2020, 10). This very much applies to the Pan-African e-Network.

36. This optimism has led to the adoption of a digital health resolution by the 71st World Health Assembly in May 2018. For an overview of the kinds of desires that are being invested in digital health, including in telehealth and telemedicine, see WHO 2005a, 2005b, 2005c, 2010; Rockefeller Foundation 2010; and Vital Wave Consulting 2012.

37. For a summary of these concerns, see Chib 2013; Huang, Blaschke, and Lucas 2017; Labrique et al. 2018; and Wilson et al. 2014.

38. Aranda-Jan, Mohutsiwa-Dibe, and Loukanova (2014); Tomlinson et al. (2013).

39. The importance of data, metrics, and evidence is a key theme in global health literature, funding, planning, and modes of intervention—including in discussions of scaling. For critical discussions, see Adams 2016; Biruk 2018; Duclos 2019a; Erikson 2019; Farman and Rottenburg 2019; Lorway 2017; Mahajan 2019; Rottenburg and Merry 2015; Storeng and Béhague 2017.

40. Interview with the author, New Delhi.

41. "What if large infrastructure projects have another relationship to time?" asks Timothy Mitchell in a recent essay (Mitchell 2020). The virtue of large infrastructure projects, suggests Mitchell, may be built not to accelerate things but to introduce a *delay* and "place the future further away" (Mitchell 2020). Infrastructure projects then appear as devices for creating a delay and stretching forward the passage of time: they "introduce an interruption, a gap, out of which the present extracts wealth from the future" (Mitchell 2020).

42. Kalam often called for the creation of "Brand India." But here I suggest that Kalam himself, as charismatic leader, personified that brand perhaps better than anyone else. As one can read in a biography displayed at the Kalam Memorial in New Delhi, "Dr. Kalam embodies the story an emerging India." See chapter 4 for more on how this was key to the affective power of PAN.

43. In contrast with most other participating African hospitals, TCIL hired local engineers to operate PAN's activities at the CHNU Fann. This was done at the request of the Senegalese government.

44. I borrow the image of India as "empire of speculation" from Bear, Birla, and Puri (2015).

45. Patients, for example, remained vexingly invisible in PAN's everyday medical operations. In the pages that follow, I have been careful not to make patients fully present but rather to show how their absence is central to PAN's promises. While making patients

whole might have helped with filling the voids in otherwise fissured stories, it might have compromised the reader's capacity to feel how absent people and things are constitutive of PAN's speculative power and thus engage with some of PAN's most troubling effects.

46. Language, notes media theorist McKenzie Wark, always "extends a little too far" as it claims to "girdle whole worlds, real or imagined" (Wark 2015, 181). Ethnographic language is certainly no exception.

1. A SHINING EXAMPLE

1. Kissinger's arrogance vis-á-vis the Global South is well documented. This particular phrase was reported by Gabriel Valdés, foreign minister of Chile, who traced it back to a conversation in 1969 in which Kissinger noted, "Mr. Minister, you made a strange speech. You come here speaking of Latin America, but this is not important. Nothing important can come from the South. History has never been produced in the South. The axis of history starts in Moscow, goes to Bonn, crosses over to Washington, and then goes to Tokyo. What happens in the South is of no importance. You're wasting your time" (Hersh 1983, 263).

2. For discussions of the role of civilizational uniqueness, or at least the perception of it, in the making of Indian foreign policy, see Abraham 2007, Singh 2019, Srinivasan 2019, or Thussu 2013.

3. In a speech given in Lok Sabha on September 17, 1955, Nehru thus summarized his views: "Peaceful co-existence is not a new idea for us in India. It has been our way of life and is as old as our thought and culture. About 2,200 years ago, a great son of India, Ashoka, proclaimed it and inscribed it on rock and stone, which exist today and give us his message. . . . In the old days, we talked of religion and philosophy; now we talk more of the economic and social system. But the approach is the same now as before" (Nehru 1961, 101).

4. Similarly, Narendra Modi, the prime minister of India as of the writing of this book (2024), rarely misses an opportunity to remind his international audiences that vasudhaiva kutumbakam stands for India's age-old belief in global integration, bridging distance and "uniting humanity" (ANI 2018). For Modi, India's contribution to the "global good" should be seen as an extension of India's ancient philosophy of vasudhaiva kutumbakam (The Hindu BusinessLine 2021). Modi's invocation of vasudhaiva kutumbakam, however, is of a different nature from Nehru's. For Modi, political claims of vasudhaiva kutumbakam are deeply entangled with a Hindu nationalist agenda. As was noted by Sangeeta Kamat, while vasudhaiva kutumbakam resonates with humanist principles of a universal humankind, "within the Hindu nationalist movement, the term refers to a political project to spread the influence of Hindu dharma (religion, customs) across the world, and to make the world a Hindu Rashtra (nation)" (Kamat 2004, 275).

5. Interview with the author, New Delhi.

6. As noted by historian Gerard McCann, the "continuities of Afro-Indian historical brotherhood have become the apparent *sine qua non* for descriptions of renewed neoliberal India-Africa relations" (McCann 2013, 260).

7. Irani and Philip (2018) show how nationalist, capitalist, and technological promises are deeply entangled in contemporary India. They therefore argue that a decolonial approach to computing, and indeed to technology, cannot rest on the celebration of difference, given how difference has become integrated into—and captured by—both the rising culture of entrepreneurship and resurgent nationalism in India.

8. For an analysis of dream-making in contemporary capitalist India, see Cross 2014.

9. For example, in *The Darker Side of Western Modernity*, Walter Mignolo suggests that decoloniality "originated among Third World Countries after the Bandung Conference in 1955, and also dispersed all over the world" (2011, xi–xii).

10. Other important meetings, although certainly less "mythical" than Bandung, in which Nehru attempted to define an "Indian" contribution to Asia-Africa cooperation

include the Asian Relations Conference which took place in New Delhi in 1947, and the Non-Aligned Conference in Belgrade in 1961.

11. Claims to cultural or scientific superiority, used as justification for colonial rule, are very well documented in many different historical contexts. See, for instance, Arnold 1993 and Metcalf 1997. As Mbembe summarizes, colonization was presented as a form of assistance, education, and moral treatment for the congenital idiocy of "indigenous peoples." Colonialism was thus conceived as "a gift of civilization" (2017, 65).

12. At the Asian Relations Conference in New Delhi on March 24, 1947, Nehru articulated his thoughts on the relationship between nationalism and humanity in these terms: "We seek no narrow nationalism. Nationalism has a place in each country and should be fostered, but it must not be allowed to become aggressive and come in the way of international development. . . . The freedom that we envisage is not to be confined to this nation or that or to a particular people, but must spread out over the whole human race. That universal human freedom cannot also be based in the supremacy of any particular class. It must be the freedom of the common man everywhere and full of opportunities for him to develop" (1947).

13. In *Nehru and Resurgent Africa*, Hari Sharan Chhabra suggests that vasudhaiva kutumbakam gained political significance in the context of the fight against imperialist expansion: "Nehru made the countries of Asia and Africa understand that if India became free, the liberation of their own countries could not be far behind. Conversely, it was well understood that the countries of Asia and Africa could never hope to throw off the foreign yoke unless India became free. Vasudhaiva Kutumbakam (the world is but a family) was one of the appropriate mottos which India's unique philosopher-statesman Dr. S. Radhakrishnan suggested when India became free. It encompassed in it what Mohandas Gandhi taught, and much more than that. The essence of this oft-repeated Sanskrit saying was reflected in Jawaharlal Nehru's life and work" (1989, 2).

14. See Final Communiqué 2009.

15. An illustration of that nostalgic storytelling can be found in Anna Tsing's *Friction*, where she associates the Bandung Conference with a space for "reclaiming the dream space of the globe"—a space of peace and freedom (Tsing 2005, 81–87).

16. Lee (2010, 12). According to Robert Vitalis, there was never a successor to the Bandung Conference, "not least because divisions of the first had been real, and no grounds for sustaining that coalition existed on the basis of color, coexistence, or neocolonialism" (2013, 278).

17. At the conclusion of the Bandung Conference, Nehru voiced his wishes for increased Asian-African cooperation by insisting that "the tragedy of Africa is greater than that of any other continent, whether it is racial or political. It is up to Asia to help Africa to the best of her ability because we are sister continents" (Nehru 1955, 291).

18. Some, like Manu Bhagavan, emphasize the fact that Nehru's dreams of wholeness, and specifically of One World, feature an indeterminacy that allowed for diversity to find its way back into a global order. Bhagavan writes, "What set One World apart, nonetheless, and reflected the truly radical nature of Indian foreign policy was the fact that the ultimate objective was not predetermined. Whereas the League of Nations saw nation states as the end product, controlled within a certain kind of European diplomatic regime, and the Comintern saw global communism as the necessary culmination of world history, Indian internationalism allowed for different people to choose different outcomes, mandating only that everyone accepts the principle of difference and that none be allowed to harm another. The units and mechanisms of One World were left unchartered, to be agreed upon only during the journey" (Bhagavan 2017, 224).

19. I am grateful to Ramah McKay for expressing this clearly when commenting on a draft version of this chapter.

20. Nehru's dedication to modern science as a means for both development and pedagogy was well summarized in his address to the Indian Science Congress in December 1937: "Politics led me to economics and this led me inevitably to science and the scientific approach to all our problems and to life itself. It was science alone that could solve these problems of hunger and poverty, of insanitation and illiteracy, of superstition and deadening custom and tradition, of vast resources turning to waste, of a rich country inhabited by starving people" (Nehru 1983, 442). For discussions of Nehru's modernist approach to science and technology, which has played a key role in shaping the idea of the nation in postcolonial India, see Arnold 2013, Nandy 1988, and Prakash 1999.

21. There is also little research documenting the circulation of cooperation and capital between India and Africa in the years after Bandung. As was noted by Dilip M. Menon, "It is interesting that in recent attempts to resuscitate the Bandung moment, there is still precious little research on actually existing connections and alignments ranging from student exchanges to technology transfer and financial assistance" (2014, 242).

22. The Colombo Plan is a regional intergovernmental organization aimed at economic development in Asia and the Pacific. As part of the South-South Technical Cooperation Scheme of the Colombo Plan, the government of India launched the Technical Cooperation Scheme (TCS), providing technical assistance to the signatories of the plan.

23. The report stated, "The assistance given by the developing countries to each other will serve not only to reduce their dependence on the assistance of the developed countries and thus make their burden a little lighter but also promote international cooperation for mutual benefit" (Government of India 1964, par. 86).

24. The Non-Aligned Movement Summit held in Cairo in 1964, as well as Indira Gandhi's African Safari in the same year, testified to the troublesome times Indo-African solidarity was going through: clearly, Indian influence had lost ground to its Chinese rival. See Dubey 1991, 37.

25. Examples include the computerization of the office of the prime minister of Senegal; assistance in the transformation of the educational system of South Africa; equipment and expertise for enhancing agricultural productivity in Ghana, Senegal, Burkina Faso, and Mali; and vocational training in small-scale industry and entrepreneurship development. Among the various sectors, IT and computing skills represent a significant share of the training made available through the program and are in high demand in recipient countries. See Beri 2003, 220, and Chand 2011 for more examples.

26. While it is essentially a bilateral scheme, the scope of ITEC's activities expanded in the 2010s to become associated with regional and multilateral organizations such as the African Union (AU), the Pan-African Parliament, the African-Asian Rural Development Organization (AARDO) and the World Trade Organisation (WTO).

27. For detailed analysis of these factors, see Bijoy 2010, Kragelund 2010, Price 2004, Sinha 2010, and Six 2009.

28. The attention paid to the African continent by major business organizations in India is suggestive in this regard. For example, out of the sixty-two working papers published by the Exim Bank of India since 2012, sixteen were specifically dedicated to expanding trade with either the whole continent or certain regions in particular.

29. This does not mean that these Indian cooperation projects all carry a commercial component. It is rather a collection of projects composing a piecemeal kind of cooperation. Recent projects include the construction of a presidential office in Ghana, the National Assembly building in Gambia, the Kosti Power plant in Sudan, water treatment projects in Tanzania, and IT parks in Mozambique and E-Swatini (Swaziland). For more on Indian projects contemporary to although of smaller scale than PAN, see Duclos 2012.

30. The Addis Ababa Declaration that emerged out of the summit was also explicit in this regard: "Africa is determined to partner in India's economic resurgence as India

is committed to be a close partner in Africa's renaissance" (Second Africa-India Forum Summit 2011).

31. Interview with the author, New Delhi.

32. Other smaller-scale examples include the declaration of an International Yoga Day (in 2015) at the United Nations and the launching of the International Solar Alliance.

33. I focus here on telemedicine networks aimed at the provision of medical care with a transnational dimension. It is important to note that telemedicine programs have been developed in different national settings for decades. Countries like Australia, Canada, Japan, and the United States all conducted telemedicine experiments in the 1980s and 1990s. It should also be noted that the provision of medical care at a distance has a much longer history. The possibility for doctors to use the telephone to ease their practice was first suggested in the correspondence section of *The Lancet* in 1879, under the rubric "Practice by Telephone" (*The Lancet* 1879). Experiments with medical consultations taking place over the telephone network, conducted by the inventor of the electrocardiograph, Wilhelm Einthoven, in the early twentieth century, are considered the early days of telemedicine. For a history of the mention of the usage of phones for medical purposes in *The Lancet* over one hundred years, see Aronson 1977. For a thorough, if uncritical, history of telemedicine, see Bashshur and Shannon 2009.

34. Operated by the Boston-based nonprofit SATELLIFE, HealthNet was launched in 1989. It used radio and satellite technology to connect health professionals around the world. In the early 2000s, it was considered the most expansive telemedicine network. HealthNet provided low-cost "store-and-forward" telemedicine services in which different types of health information—including scientific literature, messages, and image files— were being transferred (Groves 1996, Royall 1998). It did not allow real-time interaction but could provide support in the management of difficult cases. HealthNet was totally independent from international telecommunication networks, as it used its own small but dedicated packet satellite—not to be confused with PAN's geostationary communication satellite, with much higher bandwidth capacity. By the time PAN was launched, Health-Net was active in more or less twenty African countries. India was also connected, and there is some evidence that Indian doctors were using the network. In 1999, the Swinfen Charitable Trust (SCT), a UK-based charity, established low-cost telemedicine to provide specialist advice to doctors in developing countries and isolated locations. It is also an email teleconsultation system based on story-and-forward technology. By the time PAN was announced, SCT connected a dozen hospitals. The SCT is still active today. For details, see Graham et al. 2003 and Swinfen and Swinfen 2002.

35. These experiments were conducted by the Tripler Army Medical Center (TAMC), the headquarters of the Pacific Regional Medical Command of the armed forces administered by the US Army in the state of Hawaii. A telemedicine network was established as part of the Pacific Island Healthcare Project (PIHP) in 1997. It consisted of a store-and-forward system for consultation and patient referral, using email communication. The aim was apparently to provide humanitarian medical care to underserved Indigenous peoples of the USAPI at a reasonable cost. See Person 2000 for details. NASA has also been playing a key role in the early experiments of telemedicine both in the United States and globally. Starting in the 1960s, space medicine was an important component in NASA's missions. Providing support to astronauts was a key concern in a context where the effects of spaceflight on the human body were poorly understood. Space medicine was to help overcome the potential limitations of the human body in space. But it was on the Tohono O'odham reservation that NASA started to experiment with telemedicine with the launch of the Space Technology Applied to Rural Papago Health Care (STARPAHC) program in 1973. For a critical history of the programme, see Greene, Braitberg, and Bernadett 2020. For a 1995 survey of NASA's international telemedicine efforts, see Ferguson, Doarn, and Scott 1995.

36. Soon, however, telemedicine started to attract more attention and investment within development and global health spheres. Spurred by growth in bandwidth availability along with spiking cellular penetration, eHealth networks would soon be implemented all over the Global South and in sub-Saharan Africa in particular. For example, during the summer of 2008, the Rockefeller Foundation hosted a month-long conference series at its Bellagio Center on the theme of *Making the eHealth Connection: Global Partnerships, Local Solutions.* Over two hundred organizations gathered to establish an action plan aimed at facilitating the global expansion of eHealth. Participants included global health organizations such as the Bill and Melinda Gates Foundation, PEPFAR, Partners in Health, UNICEF, and the United Nations Foundation as well as large technology companies. The conference led to a report that suggested eHealth could "reverse the tide of failing health systems" and become a "great equalizer between rich and poor, healthy and ill" (Rockefeller Foundation 2010, 51). Starting in 2004, the World Health Organization published many reports on eHealth. See WHO 2004, 2005a, 2005b. Slowly, connecting the world would become a global health priority.

37. Already, when inaugurating the Indian Science Congress in 1937, Nehru summarized his technocentric vision of social development: "Politics led me to economics, and this led me inevitably to science and the scientific approach to all our problems and to life itself. It was science alone that could solve these problems of hunger and poverty, of insanitation and illiteracy, of superstition and deadening custom and tradition, of vast resources turning to waste, of a rich country inhabited by starving people" (Nehru 1983, 442). Years later, as prime minister of India, Nehru presided over the establishment of institutions such as the Atomic Energy Commission (AEC, 1948), the All India Institute of Medical Sciences (AIIMS, 1956), the Council of Scientific and Industrial Research (CSIR, 1956), the National Institutes of Technology (NIT, 1956), and the Indian Institutes of Technology (IIT, 1961).

38. As Amrita Shah notes in his biography of Sarabhai, "One of his favourite phrases was 'leapfrogging.' It referred to his great faith, along with Bhabha and Nehru, in the ability of technology to enable developing countries to circumvent the long, arduous processes followed by the Western world." See Shah 2007, 130.

39. S. K. Das summarizes the claim: "ISRO has capabilities that are comparable to the best anywhere in the world, but what makes it different is the way in which ISRO's satellites deliver services to the society, by shriking both time and distance." See Das 2007, xii; but also Harvey 2000 and Sheehan 2007.

40. ISRO has also sent nearly twenty remote sensing satellites into orbit over the past three decades. These have multiple functions related to mapping and monitoring the territory, including the prevention of natural disasters, the identification of natural resources, and the forecasting of fish stocks, among other things.

41. SITE was also supported by other international organizations such as the United Nations Development Programme (UNDP), UNESCO, UNICEF, and the International Telecommunications Union (ITU).

42. Interview with the author, Chennai.

43. A former director of telemedicine at ISRO recalled, "Apollo and Narayana, they wanted to do it and they found out that ISRO is there. They approached us. Apollo approached us. SGPGI in Lucknow was trying to do with the telecommunication lines. So we brought all major institutions to tell them: 'ISRO will provide you connectivity but you have a commitment that you will serve the rural population, wherever we decide, which state and all'" (interview with the author, Bangalore).

44. For histories of telemedicine in India written by its key actors, see Bhaskaranarayan, Satyamurthy, and Remilla 2009; Ganapathy and Ravindra 2009; and Mishra, Singh, and Chand 2012.

45. A former director of satellite communication services at ISRO explained to me, "Our idea is to experiment this with the people who are unreached. We also in the beginning never thought about an economic model. We only looked at the social cost. So most of the cost for this equipment was by ISRO. The only thing is whoever partnered with us, we wanted them to do free service. No user fees. All those people with whom we have partnered, even if they have a profit motive, they were willing to do this. Those are the people with whom we have partnered. . . . For example, Sankara Nethrayalaya, Apollo, Fortis. They cross subsidize. If there is a revenue in their mind, we are not part of it" (interview with the author, Bangalore).

46. As such, telemedicine reflects the growing importance in India of corporate social responsibility and public-private partnerships. It also speaks to a cultural and political sensibility according to which corporate work is narrated in socially beneficial terms (Irani 2019), and "pro-poor pro-market" development projects are being advertised as technical solutions to complex societal problems (Chakravartty 2012). This "culture of corporate intervention" is particularly present in ICT spheres (Sarkar 2017).

47. Prof. S. K. Mishra, pioneer of telemedicine in India, thus explained how a social model could also be seen as a business model: "The private sector won't run at loss. They try to partner with government projects. Somebody is paying for infrastructure, somebody is paying for bandwidth and, of course, you are giving free consultations but at the same time you achieve your own business platform to bring in new patients. That's what they're doing. Quite wise. See what the government job is? It is to see that people get access to health care. Whether within the public health system or the private sector. Government is facilitating, for connecting, for giving access" (interview with the author, Lucknow).

48. For discussions of the impact of the reforms on health care, see Lefebvre 2010; Qadeer 2000, 27; Sen 2001.

49. These agreements were later heavily criticized as it became clear that corporate hospitals rarely complied. Harsh words about such agreements can be found in a report by the Public Accounts Committee on the granting of land to private hospitals at a discount: "Ultimately, what was started with a grand idea of benefiting the poor turned out to be a hunting ground for the rich in the garb of public charitable institutions" (Public Accounts Committee 2005, 26).

50. Interview with the author, Bangalore.

51. A manager at Fortis Healthcare and pioneer of the corporate hospital sector in India explained, "There are no payers [in rural areas]. If you were a shareholder for Fortis, would you allow me to open something there? You won't! The corporates have their own answerability to their shareholders" (interview with the author, New Delhi).

52. Dr. Devi Shetty, cardiac surgeon and the chairman of Narayan Hrudayalaya, a leading hospital in the telemedicine in India, explains, "In terms of disease management, there is [a] 99% possibility that the person who is unwell does not require [an] operation. If you don't operate, you don't need to touch the patient. And if you don't need to touch the patient, you don't need to be there. You can be anywhere, since the decision on healthcare management is based on history and interpretation of images . . . so technically speaking, 99% of health-care problems can be managed by the doctors staying at a remote place— linked by telemedicine" (Bagchi 2006).

53. This is a narrative that is not unique to India, nor is it always mobilized in parochial ways. In an interview in which he discussed the potential effects of the internet on the African continent, Achille Mbembe also mobilized the precolonial past as evidence of an African cultural world particularly suited for the internet age: "In fact the world of Africa, the pre-colonial world, as well as the world of now, has always been somewhat digital. And what we see now is the reconciliation of that culture and a form that is coming from outside. . . . The idea is that Africa was digital before the digital. And when you study the

cultural history of the continent carefully, a number of things come to the fore in terms of how African societies have constituted themselves and how they operated. . . . This flexibility and this capacity for constant innovation, extension of the possible, that is also the spirit of the Internet, it is the spirit of the digital, and it is the same spirit you will find in pre-colonial and contemporary Africa" (Mbembe and van der Haak 2015). I discuss this question in more detail in chapter 4.

2. MEDICINE FROM THE AIR

1. In addition to teleconsultations themselves, Indian doctors sometimes share scientific publications to which Fann's doctors may not have access. It is not uncommon for a Fann doctor to ask Indian colleagues if they would share articles or references related to a particular case. Sometimes, articles are attached to a patient's file. Given the prohibitive cost of subscribing to scientific journals, access to literature is not straightforward at Fann. Clinicians sometimes use a service offered by the Agence universitaire de la francophonie, where articles can be found for them for a fee. Sometimes, one of the doctors goes on an internship in a country and comes back with a code to access scientific journals that he can share with his colleagues for a while. Also, it is sometimes possible to have access to some journals at Cheikh-Anta-Diop University. But the choices are limited, and you have to travel to do the research.

2. Reaching out for colleagues outside of the physical walls of the hospital is common practice in medicine. But the possibilities to do so have proliferated with digital health. In the *New York Times* column "Diagnosis," Dr. Lisa Sanders speaks thusly of the crowdsourcing of medical diagnosis enabled by digital technology: "Getting the right diagnosis is the most important thing you can do for a patient. . . . One of the tools that doctors use are the other doctors in the room. And whether you're going to get a diagnosis or not really depends on who's in that room and who might see something that they recognize and understand, and then identify it. So what we're doing is just making the room that much bigger. More people, more experience."

3. My understanding of the work of engineers is informed by a growing amount of ethnographic studies that have paid attention to work on maintenance and repair. This includes work by Denis and Pontille (2015), Graham and Thrift (2007), Henke (2000), and Martínez and Laviolette (2019). For research focusing on information and communication technology (ICT), see Callén and Criado (2016) and Jackson, Pompe, and Krieshok (2012). Drawing upon Denis (2019, 284), it is possible to suggest that paying attention to these engineers' work invites us to shift attention from processes of design and "form giving" to those of maintenance and "form-keeping."

4. Interview with the author, Dakar.

5. Interview with the author, Dakar.

6. Interview with the author, Dakar.

7. Interview with the author, Dakar.

8. Indian medical specialists are paid for their participation in PAN. According to the information I obtained, they are paid between 1,000 and 1,500 rupees per hour, or between US\$20 and US\$30. By comparison, a consultation in person with a specialist at an Apollo hospital would cost between 500 and 1,000 rupees.

9. With the exception of the electronic medical record system (confidential), there is no registry of all PAN teleconsultation cases. Each hospital keeps a history of its activities, but I have not always had access to it. It is difficult for me to draw quantitative conclusions about the types of cases seen, diagnoses made, and so on. So I rely on the teleconsultations I have witnessed, some of the documents that have been made available to me, and conversations with engineers and physicians.

10. Dr. Leye explains, "The more patients you deal with, the more experience you have, the more you get to see rare things. They're in hyper-specialized centers, where they get a

lot of cases. So they have some experience with rare cases. We most often call on them for these cases. The rare cases or the difficult ones" (interview with the author, Dakar).

11. This situation gave rise to a huge misunderstanding. Although Dr. Leye had requested the presence of a surgeon, the teleconsultation took place with a cardiologist. Yet months after the event, Dr. Leye still believed that Dr. Ambedkar was a surgeon. Since it was not the first teleconsultation between Dr. Leye and Dr. Ambedkar, it's hard to understand the scope of the confusion. In light of my discussions with Dr. Leye, it is my understanding that he had always believed that his interlocutor was either a surgeon or a cardiologist with surgical training, or at least that he had consulted a fellow surgeon before presenting himself for teleconsultation. In one way or another, this was not the case. Nevertheless, Dr. Ambedkar's explanations seemed to have satisfied Fann's medical specialists.

12. The fact that Mamadou was not Senegalese was not a key factor since even for Senegalese citizens, the cost of medical treatment is not fully assumed by the state and can be prohibitive. Under such conditions, it is not uncommon for a patient or family to take several weeks to find the necessary amount before returning to the service, even if the treatment is urgent. In other cases, patients never come back.

13. Such humanitarian logic has been the object of repeated criticism over the years. Criticism tends to insist on the fact that the transport of patients can be prohibitively expensive, can come with high levels of distress—especially for children traveling without family members—and, above all, can reproduce a dependence on foreign aid instead of developing the medical infrastructure required to take care of the patients locally (Brousse et al. 2003; Leblanc 2009; Razgallah 2019).

14. Scholarly literature also documents the limitations and shortcomings of such short humanitarian missions. Leblanc summarizes, "A short mission may not have enough time to train local doctors in complicated surgical techniques. The host hospital may not have the equipment and money to maintain a program. The health care professionals may not have enough time for training to build a program, often complicated by language barriers. Most organizations can only fund a few missions per year and relatively few children can be treated with each visit while the intentions for sustainability is not realized" (Leblanc 2009, 90).

15. It should be noted that the DTCS was launched with the support of various international institutions and NGOs including the Japan International Cooperation Agency and La Chaîne de l'Espoir itself.

16. Interview with the author, Dakar.

17. Interview with the author, Dakar.

18. These patterns are evidently not homogenous across the African continent. For example, the routes for the circulation of patients between Mauritius or East Africa and India are already much better established. Chapter 4 examines how PAN contributed to this.

19. This also applies to telemedicine. Social science research has shown that telemedicine networks do not operate from a blank slate. In spite of the frequent framing of digital health in terms of flow, transmission, and mobility, there is no erasure of distance and place in everyday work. For ethnographic work, see Mort, Finch, and May 2009; Oudshoorn 2012; Pols 2012; and Sánchez-Criado et al. 2014.

20. On the highway between Dakar and Thiès, one can see a large antenna in the shape of a parabola: It is the Gandoul communication Earth Station. With a diameter of thirty meters, it was the first of its kind in Africa. The Gandoul antenna was built in 1970 and inaugurated by President Senghor in 1972. The antenna first brought public television to Senegal. Then, in the early 1980s, the antenna would be central to a collaboration between NASA and Senegal as the Gandoul station was selected as a control and communications station for the Space Shuttle *Columbia*. While it is no longer in operation, the antenna

is widely recognized as part of the telecommunications heritage in Senegal and also in Africa. To this day, it has remained the source of significant local pride in Senegal.

21. Interview with the author, Addis Ababa.

22. Although I could not find confirmation of this in any institutional document of the projects, a high-ranking officer involved from the early days of the project mentioned that at the very beginning a satellite from Eutelsat was also momentarily used for the pilot phase of the project—before Rascom-QAF1 was launched.

23. The launch of the Regional African Satellite Communication Organisation was itself created in 1992. The Pan-African space initiatives took almost two decades to become operational. RASCOM's satellite operations are managed by RascomStar, a private company registered in Mauritius.

24. RASCOM's mission statement reads like this: "RASCOM's mission is to design, implement, operate and maintain the space segment of the African telecommunications satellite system and translate into services and tools for African integration, all the opportunities provided by satellites by linking it, where necessary, with any other appropriate technology." See http://www.rascom.org.

25. As was suggested by RascomStar's CEO at the launch of the Rascom-QAF1 satellite (the predecessor of Rascom-QAF1R) in 2007, "All Africans are happy to share this historic moment with us. Rascom-QAF1 will help bridge the digital divide between Africa and the rest of the world. It will save us hundreds of millions of dollars that are now spent on international operators" (Le Monde 2007; translation is mine).

26. Interview with the author, Dakar.

27. An officer at the African Union Commission explained, "But the only fault I really have with it, which is actually correctable in the end, is the quality of the network in terms of the capacity it provides. If we had put a 512 kbps carrier instead of 384 kbps, we might have had a better quality, but we would have invested more. So in their design, the Indians have adjusted to the quality-price factor, a minimum of quality with a lower price" (interview with the author, Dakar).

28. Interview with the author, Dakar.

29. Interview with the author, Dakar.

30. Interview with the author, Dakar.

31. Before TCIL took the lead of the project, ISRO was very much involved in drafting the early plans for PAN. According to many scientists interviewed while preparing this book, the recent history of ISRO's work on telemedicine in India—and its overall philosophy of "space technology in the service of humankind"—was instrumental in making satellites a key component of PAN. In fact, it is quite plausible that without ISRO's active engagement in telemedicine, PAN would not have been imagined or deemed possible.

32. This is not always obvious. Indian corporate hospitals are obviously already connected by fiber optics. However, it is not always through Bharti Airtel. One hospital manager thus criticized the company's monopoly on PAN connectivity. His hospital was located in an area not served by Bharti Airtel and had to wait months for the connection to be established. During this time, the hospital could not participate in PAN.

33. The servers were mainly storing tele-education data. For reasons of medical confidentiality, the project's telemedicine activities were not stored at the data center but rather at each participating hospital—more on this later.

34. ATLANTIS-2 was preceded by a few submarine cables. Already, in the mid-1970s, Sonatel (the country's sole telephone operator at the time) benefited from the Antinea and Fraternity submarine cables. The former connected Dakar to Casablanca while the latter connected Dakar to Abidjan. These were not digital cables but analog cables, however. ATLANTIS-1, installed after Antinea and Fraternity, was also an analog cable.

35. In her brilliant ethnography of undersea cables, Starosielski (2015) suggests that we challenge our imagination of networks as immaterial, distributed flow by making visible the physicality, topography, and history of the lines between network nodes. She writes, "Although our digital environment appears to be a space of mobility, radically changing every few years, the backbone for the global Internet continues to be sunk along historical and political lines, tending to reinforce existing global inequalities" (Starosielski 2015, 12).

36. ATLANTIS-2 (2000) and SAT-3/WASC (2002) provided high-speed, high-band-width links between Europe and fourteen countries on the west coast of Africa while SAFE (2002) connected Mauritius, Réunion, and South Africa to India and Malaysia. Source: https://www.submarinecablemap.com.

37. These include Seacom (2009), Lion (2009), Teams (2009), MainOne (2010), EASSy (2010), Glo1 (2011), WACS (2012), and the giant ACE (2012), which on its own is connecting more than 450 million people. This proliferation of undersea cables is widely touted as an engine for bridging the digital divide and fostering economic growth. At the time of writing, two of the world's biggest technology companies, Google and Facebook, are building new undersea internet cable systems that will bring bandwidth—namely, Equiano (Google) and 2Africa (with Facebook as cofounder). However, it should be noted that a majority of these networks are not owned or operated by African stakeholders. SEA-COM is a notable exception: The 17,000 km submarine cable connecting South Africa, Kenya, Tanzania, Mozambique, Djibouti, France, and India is 75 percent African owned, although the segment of SEACOM connecting to India is owned by Tata Communications.

38. DICOM stands for Digital Imaging and Communications in Medicine.

39. According to Ashoka, setting up a site cost about US$500,000.

40. Medical equipment was supplied by Recorders and Medicare Systems Pvt, ORG Informatics Limited, and TBL International Limited (co-owned by TCIL). All these suppliers were Indian companies.

41. The UPS were of the Numeric (Indian company) brand, and the model was Digital HPE 1150.

42. Anthropologists and STS scholars have insisted for some time on the need to pay better attention to the invisible but also boring labor that supports infrastructures on an everyday basis. See, for example, Star 1999 and Van Eijk 2018.

43. Two years before the initial publication of *The Birth of the Clinic*, Foucault wrote about the Renaissance madman in these terms: "He is put in the interior of the exterior, and inversely . . . he is a prisoner in the midst of what is the freest, the openest of routes: bound fast at the infinite crossroads" (Foucault [2001] 1961, 9).

44. Foucault will later regret his usage of the notion of "gaze" (*le regard*) in *The Birth of the Clinic* (Foucault 1973). This notion, he thought, could give the impression of reducing the "gaze" to the sense of sight. By contrast, as Gilles Deleuze later notes in his inspired reading of Foucault, "visibilities are neither the acts of a seeing subject nor the data of a visual meaning" (Deleuze 1988, 59). The notion of "gaze" could suggest a relationship between a fully constituted subject and an objective exterior field. The "medical gaze" does not refer to a knowing subject exposing a truth that has hitherto been hidden from science but rather to a peculiar form of perceptual problematization.

45. Grégoire Chamayou thus summarizes this notion of copresence in his brilliant examination of drone warfare and remote killing: "The problem is that what we call 'distance' covers several dimensions that are confused in our ordinary experience but which technologies both disaggregate and redistribute spatially. So it is now possible to be both close and distant, according to dimensions that are unequal and that combine a pragmatic co-presence. Physical distance no longer necessarily implies perceptual distance" (Chamayou 2015, 116).

46. To be able to repeat, suggests Wendy Hui Kyong Chun, "is the basis of connection, or the basis of the elucidation/imagining of connection. To be able to repeat is what links the machinic and the human" (Chun 2015, 300).

47. Bowker and Star defined articulation as "a work done in real time to manage contingencies: work that get things back on track in the face of the unexpected, that modifies action to accommodate unanticipated contingencies" (Bowker and Star 1999, 310). For a good summary of articulation work with special attention to computer-supported cooperative work (CSCW), see Star and Strauss 1999.

3. THE ARCHIPELAGO OF CARE

1. The names of all doctors in chapter 3 were changed to ensure confidentiality.

2. "NEWUSER" stands for Dr. Daar, while "APOLLO_CHENNAI-Dr.PC-03" stands for Dr. Mohan.

3. The cost is in Indian rupees. In USD, it converts to more or less $600 for the endoscopy and $300 for the CT scan.

4. Dr. Mohan, gastroenterologist, Apollo Hospital, interview with the author, Chennai.

5. This is a narrative that I have also encountered in Senegal. According to a cardiologist at Fann, "At the hospital level, now in India we are working in relatively modern hospitals, but at a certain time, in a relatively recent period, they have been in the same problems as us. So they knew how to adapt. The developed countries had at one time the same problems as here, but it goes back a long time! While, on the other hand, India is not yet at the level of the developed countries, they have had the same problems as us in a shorter timeframe than in the developed countries. So it's easier for these people to share their experience, how they did to adapt when they had these problems and they did not have the means they have now. We feel it in the interactions because they have the same problems as us! In their speech, we feel that they know" (interview with the author, Dakar).

6. The notion that telemedicine could be a promising venue for South-South collaboration predates PAN. In fact, a few months before PAN was announced, Geissbuhler et al. thus summarized this potential: "A promising perspective is the fostering, through decentralized collaborative networks, of South-South exchanges of expertise. For example, there is neurosurgical expertise in Dakar, Senegal, which is a neighboring country to Mali. A tele-consultation between these two countries would make sense for two reasons: a) physicians in Senegal understand the context of Mali much better than those from northern countries, and b) a patient requiring neurosurgical treatment would most likely be treated in Dakar rather than in Europe" (Geissbuhler et al. 2003, 252).

7. Dr. Faye, interview with the author, Dakar.

8. Dr. Sow, interview with the author, Dakar.

9. For discussions of the globalization of Indian hospitals, see Bärnreuther 2021, Baru 2018, Bochaton and Lefebvre 2008, Kumar 2015, and Lefebvre 2010.

10. Medical tourism is a concept that aims—but probably fails—to encompass a wide variety of transnational mobilities through which patients seek treatment. Anthropologists have done a fine job of documenting its multiple dimensions. See, for instance, special issues of *Anthropology & Medicine* (Naraindas and Bastos 2011), *Body & Society* (Roberts and Scheper-Hughes 2011), and *Anthropologie & Santé* (Mulot, Musso, and Sakoyan 2011). See also Kaspar, Walton-Roberts, and Bochaton 2019.

11. While obtaining a visa to seek treatment in the United States or in Europe can be very difficult, visas to India can be issued within a week (Rao 2017).

12. It should be noted, however, that these are not official numbers and that numbers can vary significantly among reports.

13. Although this is a relatively common slogan, I take it specifically from Modi (2010, 128). As a manager at Manipal Hospital, a corporate tertiary care hospital in Bangalore, explained, "We are very proud. Because we are able to deliver the quality health care at a price which is 1/10 or 1/20 of the rest of the world" (Dr. Nair, interview with the author, Bangalore). This discourse is widespread. Entrepreneurs and managers within the Indian hospital sector would emphasize to me that the quality of the health care provided in their hospital is equivalent to the top institutions in the world.

14. Devi Shetty, founder and CEO of Narayana Hrudayalaya, embodies better than anyone else this "caring" dimension of Indian health care. In his own words: "India is privileged as a nation to have the largest number of medical personnel in the world, who also strive towards the service of humanity so passionately. We are certain that India will be the first country in the world to dissociate healthcare from affluence" (Narayana Hrudayalaya Healthcity 2011, 2).

15. See, for example, Kithuure 2014 or Mogaka, Mupara, and Tsoka-Gwegweni 2017. In 2015, the World Bank estimated that the African continent lost over US$1 billion a year on medical tourism abroad as it "exported money and patients to the East, especially India." Khama Rogo of the World Bank explains, "The Indian private sector is enjoying the benefits of sickness from the African continent. Young people in Africa have instead started clinics as conveyor belts for Indian clinics. 25% of the passenger loads on major airlines Kenya Airways and Ethiopian Airlines are medical tourists" (IMTJ 2016).

16. For an overview of this expansion, see Modi 2011. Of particular importance is the notion that Indian hospitals possess expertise not only in patient care but also in building hospital infrastructure and managing health care at a large scale and that this expertise in particular should be exported to Africa. According to David Rasquinha, managing director and chief executive officer of the Export-Import Bank of India, Indian cooperation with Africa in the health care sector should primarily take the form of tied aid in which concessional loans would be used to set up tertiary hospitals in African cities. Operating a tertiary hospital, Rasquinha notes in a report dedicated to the issue, is a highly skilled enterprise that "cannot be learned overnight" (Rasquinha 2016, 20). According to Rasquinha, the design, construction, operation, and maintenance of these hospitals would be assumed by large Indian hospital groups such as Apollo Hospitals and Fortis Healthcare, who would benefit from developing "goodwill and brand recognition at no capital cost" (21): "Twinning India's hospital construction expertise with its hospital administration expertise will be a focused, win-win approach for the Africa-India bilateral" (20).

17. As Elrod and Fortenberry describe it, the "hub-and-spoke organization design is a model which arranges service delivery assets into a network consisting of an anchor establishment (hub) which offers a full array of services, complemented by secondary establishments (spokes) which offer more limited service arrays, routing patients needing more intensive services to the hub for treatment" (Elrod and Fortenberry 2017, 26). Porter and Lee (2013) further suggest that the hub-and-spoke model, with the establishment of satellite facilities and the circulation of expertise and patients, is the primary form taken by the geographic expansion of health care providers. From an historical perspective, the recommendation to resort to a hierarchical system linking center and periphery in the distribution of health care, which is likely the legitimate ancestor of the hub-and-spoke model, is often traced back to a report published by the British Ministry of Health in 1920. The "Interim Report on the Future Provision of Medical and Allied Services" is commonly referred to as the "Dawson Report" after the name of its author, Sir Bertrand Dawson.

18. Speaking of the hub-and-spoke model, Govindarajan and Ramamurti argue that "Indian hospitals, doctors, and administrators have traditionally looked to the West for advances in medical knowledge, but it's time for the West looked to India for innovations

in health care delivery" (2013, 7) For a discussion of the hub-and-spoke expansion of Indian hospitals, see Devarakonda 2016.

19. S. K. Mishra, SGPGIMS Lucknow, interview with the author, Lucknow.

20. Project manager, Narayana Hrudayalaya Health City, interview with the author, Bangalore.

21. As Ferguson noted, the language of "flow" is a "poor metaphor for the point-to-point connectivity and networking of enclaves that confront us when we examine Africa's experience of globalization" (Ferguson 2006, 47).

22. Warwick Anderson (2014) suggested that imagining "global health" as the product of unleashed flows and circulations conceals the struggles and radical alterity implicated in scale-making. As Dilger and Mattes have also noted, anthropologists and social scientists have "exposed how profoundly the mobilities and connectivities constituting the landscaping of Global Health are shaped by transnational power relations" (Dilger and Mattes 2018, 266). Other work that has contributed to exposing these power relations, some of which are cited by Dilger and Mattes, include Brada 2011; Dilger, Kane, and Langwick 2012; and Geissler 2014.

23. As explained by Pradeep Menon (2022), in a hub-and-spoke model "the hub governs the spokes and ensures that the spoke domain follows the prescribed governance framework created by the hub domain."

24. According to an official at the Africa Union Commission, security was a key reason why the option of using a regular internet connection was rejected: "The Internet puts the project in a rather open situation, exposed to data leakage. Which is personal data. It's very difficult, people are not encouraged to know that their personal data is flowing on the Internet" (interview with the author). An engineer in charge of the PAN operations in Africa (Hub Center) explained further: "Security is being taken care of by various methods. Every site, due to this infrastructure, is having its own specific azimuth and elevation angle to look into the Rascom satellite. A technician has been positioning everything properly. That is one point. Next, everything is encrypted in the modem, which is connected to the satellite. This has to come from the hub. No one else can do it. They don't know what frequency is working. No other modem. So we are always having the numbers monitored. Unless the authorized VSAT is there, if other VSATs come we can find out. We will not permit them because they have to come through us [the Hub center]" (interview with the author).

25. Interview with the author, New Delhi.

26. Media scholars have shown how connectivity is actively engineered. As Van Dijck (2013, 152) has suggested, this engineering negotiates between "owners, users, content producers, lawmakers, engineers and marketers about the control of data and technology" (Van Dijck 2013, 152).

27. The hub-and-spoke topology is not limited to computer networks. Hub-and-spoke topologies are commonly used in fields where centralization and ease of management are important. This includes telecommunications (to route telephone and internet traffic through central hubs), logistics (e.g., to route cargo through central hubs), and supply chain management (for routing goods through central hubs for storage and distribution). Hub-and-spoke topologies are perhaps best known for their usage in the airline industry. In fact, the creation of the hub-and-spoke topology in the 1970s and 1980s is considered a key development in the airline industry, with the routing of flights through a central hub which allowed for efficient use of aircraft and easy management of flight schedules. Finally, hub-and-spoke topology is frequently found in maritime network design and extractive industries, among others.

28. Due to the time difference between Dakar and Chennai (Dakar time is five and a half hours behind Chennai), if a Dakar engineer sent a teleconsultation request in the

afternoon (Dakar time), his colleague in Chennai would take notice of it the next morning. If the teleconsultation was to take place the same day, this left only until the middle of the afternoon (morning in Dakar) to organize the appointment. This was not always obvious since it was already 2:00 p.m. (Chennai time) when the engineer in Senegal arrived at work. Both engineers thus had only a few hours to make an appointment and prepare the teleconsultation.

29. Physician, CHNU, interview with the author, Dakar.

30. Dr. Diop, CHNU Fann, interview with the author, Dakar.

31. "The most interesting part, which can allow us to see further, is the type of human relations that this can create and that will allow, for example, to boost other forms of cooperation. That's what's important. I believe that the fact that he [the Indian doctor] is here in front of me, that he calls me by my first name and I call him by his first name, if tomorrow we met in a conference that would take place in New York or in Paris, it would change a lot of things, a priori. Politicians can decide things, they can even set up frameworks. The framework was not made for that! . . . Now, what the people who use it will do with it is what is important" (Dr. Sow, CHNU Fann, interview with the author, Dakar).

32. Physician, CHNU Fann, interview with the author, Dakar.

33. This perspective is often traced back to Marx himself and his discussion of human labor as an activity by which humans effect a change of form in inert materials. The exceptional status of the human laborer is most eloquently illustrated in *Capital*: "A spider conducts operations that resemble those of a weaver, and a bee puts to shame many an architect in the construction of her cells. But what distinguishes the worst architect from the best of bees is this, that the architect raises his structure in imagination before he erects it in reality. At the end of every labour-process, we get a result that already existed in the imagination of the labourer at its commencement" (Marx [1906] 1867), 198; *Capital* vol. 1, pt. 3, ch. 7, §2). This famous example shows how, for Marx, the mental representation of an end to be achieved constitutes an essential condition for production. If this capacity to project oneself in time allows Marx to posit the uniqueness of human labor, it nonetheless has the effect of introducing a form of ahistorical exteriority, a principle of transcendental causality into the very act of production. However, how can we reconcile the fact that historical consciousness is only an artifact of material life (as Marx also posited) with this idea of an end-product already present in the imagination of the laborer? Overall, the tension that runs through Marx's work between production as an open-ended process on the one hand and construction as the actualization of a finite potential on the other poses a fundamental question: how can production be freed from the linear causality of productivism?

34. Key writings of Ingold on the topic include Ingold 2006, 2007, and 2011.

35. Ingold uses the hub-and-spoke model as an example, comparing it to the figure of the knot: "My concern is not to unravel the knot, but to compare it to the hub-and-spokes model with which I began this section (see Figure 3.8). In this latter model the hub, as a container for life, is clearly distinguished from the individuals it contains—each represented by a mobile dot—as well as from the lines connecting it to other hubs in the network. The knot, by contrast, does not contain life but is rather formed of the very lines along which life is lived. These lines are bound together in the knot, but they are not bound by it. To the contrary they trail beyond it, only to become caught up with other lines in other knots. Together they make up what I have called a meshwork. Every place, then, is a knot in the meshwork, and the threads from which it is traced are lines of wayfaring" (Ingold 2007, 100).

36. See Jackson 2018. Others have insisted that they are not so "new" as they are ignorant of other non-Western thinking. Tompkins (2016), for instance, writes, "among others, First Nations and Indigenous peoples; those humans who have never been quite human enough, as explored for instance, in postcolonial and revolutionary black thought; to some

strands of feminist thinking, for instance, de Beauvoir's thinking about the objecthood of women; and to other non-Western medical and spiritual modalities."

37. For Sloterdijk, spheres are the spaces where people live, where the average human destiny is fulfilled. Being-in-the-world means being-in-spheres. At an existential level, Sloterdijk imagines spheres as media: as membranes that mediate our relationship to the world, protecting us from perishing of immediacy or "falling into things"—the title of a paper I wrote about the ontological anthropology developed by Sloterdijk over the course of three decades. See Duclos 2019b.

38. As Bruno Latour suggested, Sloterdijk is a philosopher of design. Latour approached Sloterdijk's philosophy of design in relation to his broader post-phenomenological writings on being-in-the-world as being-in-space. Playing around with the Heideggerian notion of Dasein, he wrote, "When we say 'Dasein is *in* the world' we usually pass very quickly on the little preposition 'in.' Not Sloterdijk. In what? he asks, and in where? Are you in a room? In an air-conditioned amphitheater? And if so what sort of air pumps and energy sources keep it up?" (Latour 2008, 7). Sloterdijk's oeuvre indeed revolves around this question of the design of interior spaces but also of the conditions of viability of atmospheres. For a good overview, see Sloterdijk 2009, 2012.

39. For an analysis of Sloterdijk's spherology in relation to anthropological theories of circulation and exchange, see Povinelli 2011.

40. The actual forms taken by spheres are obviously historically shaped. For example, Sloterdijk is at time highly critical of the thesis of the "global village" developed by media theorist Marshall McLuhan. Remember McLuhan's vision in *Understanding Media*: "Today, after more than a century of electric technology, we have extended our central nervous system itself in a global embrace, abolishing both space and time as far as our planet is concerned." (McLuhan 2003, 19) Put roughly, Sloterdijk suspects McLuhan of reintroducing the theological motif of communion as a mode of being-together in the electronic age. According to Sloterdijk, the global village as envisioned by McLuhan would be driven by a kind of electronic Catholicism, illustrating the image of a fully rounded globe that must be challenged. Hence his concept of "foam," emphasizing a conception of life as multiperspectivist and heterarchic deployment. In other words, the fact that the "world has no more exterior," made explicit when the first satellites were put into orbit (more on this in chapter 4), does not mean that everyone inhabits its "interior space" under the same symbolic, economic and biopolitical conditions.

4. THE EMPIRE OF SPECULATION

1. Quote taken from: http://www.youtube.com/watch?v=n8AIC_KZ5rw. Accessed June 24, 2024.

2. Since his passing in 2015, President Kalam's ambitions for ISRO's space program have shown no sign of abating. These ambitions were on full display on August 23, 2023, when India's Chandrayaan-3 spacecraft accomplished a successful lunar landing. This made India the fourth country globally, following the United States, the USSR, and China, to achieve this milestone. State investment in costly, spectacular space missions, however, has been the object of criticism in India, underlining the gap between such expenditures and the great discrimination and poverty simultaneously faced by millions of Indians. Investigative journalist Vidya Krishnan, for instance, suggested that Chandrayaan-3 was India's own "Whitey on the moon" moment, a reference to African American Gil Scott-Heron's poem, published as a virulent critique of the Apollo mission, a project for white America while so many African Americans lived under conditions of structural racism and great poverty. Krishnan writes, "As Indian scientists—mostly upper caste, prosperous and secure in their place in the country—were celebrating the moon landing, millions of mar-

ginalized, disfranchised, impoverished Indians were suffering immensely. . . . India made it to the moon, but Indian people are still poor, still hungry. Indian women are still unsafe. No scientific triumph can obscure the degradation of human life in our country. A journey to the moon cannot hide the ever-deepening inequality and seemingly endless injustices devastating minorities" (Krishnan 2024). In my research on PAN, at times I heard versions (although generally milder in tone) of this argument as well as counterarguments.

3. As the next chapter will make even more evident, the "view from above" that accompanies satellite form in PAN comes with concrete consequences. I therefore share Lisa Stevenson's insight that deconstructing form does not mean we can neglect its efficacy: "I agree with these anthropologists of bureaucracy that things are always messier, more complicated, and more interesting 'on the ground' and that bureaucracy cannot be reduced to its ideal type. I am also sympathetic to Haraway's suggestion that we need to continually deconstruct the view from nowhere as the most faithful representation of the world at large. However, in this book I want to argue that there is a difference between reducing something (in this case bureaucracy) to its ideal type and recognizing the efficacy of its form (Kohn 2013), which in this case involves the reproduction and circulation of a view from nowhere" (Stevenson 2014, 193).

4. Dr. Kalam didn't move very far when he stepped down after five years as president of the republic on July 25, 2007. His new residence was indeed located near the presidential mansion of Rashtrapati Bhavan, in the heart of the luxurious Lutyens Bungalow Zone (LBZ). In spite of Dr. Kalam's reputation of living a rather spartan lifestyle, his new residence had been selected and fully renovated and furnished to meet the demands of its famous occupant, including the conversion of the upper part of the house into a library and reading area.

5. The primary reason I wanted to meet Kalam was obvious: He was, I had heard so many times, the visionary behind PAN. But doing fieldwork within India's telemedicine sector also led to Kalam in many ways. In the early years of PAN, and especially between 2010 and 2012, I visited dozens of telemedicine centers in India. All located within Indian hospitals, some of these were connected to PAN, and others were providing telemedicine services to other regions within India. In most if not all of these centers, there was a picture of Kalam, and stories about the president were told. I had also become acquainted with many people who were close to Kalam—including his biographer and cowriter but also scientists who had worked with him when he was president. On many occasions, the prospect of my meeting with the former president had been mentioned. Ultimately, however, it is evident to me that the background to any explanation on how I got to meet with Kalam lay in the most obvious fact: I was an educated white man doing research in India.

6. Admiration for Kalam has obviously carried on after he passed, materializing in several sites of commemoration. For example, the Dr. A. P. J. Abdul Kalam National Memorial was built in his hometown of Rameswaram, off the coast of Tamil Nadu. The memorial was designed and constructed by the Defence Research and Development Organisation (DRDO), where Kalam had spent the bulk of his career, and displays replicas of rockets and missiles that he worked on. It was inaugurated by Prime Minister Narendra Modi in 2017. Another memorial honoring Kalam was built in New Delhi. Then, the house in which Kalam grew up in Rameshwaram was converted into a museum that pays tribute to Kalam by displaying pictures, books, writings, and other personal items and artifacts that belonged to him. A military missile research center in Hyderabad was named after the "missile man" of India. Finally, Aurangzeb Road in New Delhi was renamed Dr. A. P. J. Abdul Kalam Road. These are just some examples, as there may be many more tributes to Kalam that I am not aware of.

7. Guha (2012) explains this discrepancy by insisting that Kalam was widely seen as a "good Muslim"—namely, a prominent Muslim who stood by his motherland and swore to "bomb Pakistan if circumstances so demanded." Kalam indeed occupied a unique posi-

tion within Indian politics. Although a Muslim himself, he was nominated for president by an alliance of Hindu nationalist parties led by the Bharatiya Janata Party (BJP). Because of his high popularity, the Indian National Congress also supported his candidacy. A vegetarian and a bachelor, Kalam liked to quote both Muslim and Hindu scriptures, especially the Bhagavad Gita. But it was mainly his status as the architect of India's nuclear program that earned him the admiration of nationalists, including Hindu nationalists. It is possible to suggest that Kalam tempered a radical Hindu nationalism—which claimed Vedic glory to justify ethnic segregation—with a more unifying Indian nationalism. Hence in *Ignited Minds*: "Why can't we develop a cultural—not religious—context for our heritage that serves to make Indians of us all? The time has come for us to stop differentiating. What we need today is a vision for the nation which can bring unity" (Kalam 2003, 115–16). It is also noteworthy that although he was nominated by the BJP, Kalam announced PAN a few months after the 2004 India general election, which saw the BJP lose to the Indian National Congress (INC), which would remain in power until 2014. However, Kalam always remained the BJP's candidate, as was made evident in the presidential election in 2012. Even though opinion polls still showed great popular support for Kalam, and the BJP still supported him, Kalam decided against running for reelection for lack of support from the United Progressive Alliance (UPA), led by the INC.

8. I borrow from William Mazzarella's analysis of Donald Trump's charisma: "To say that Trump-fans enjoy Trump is also to say that they enjoy themselves in him" (2022, 3).

9. Dr. Abdul Kalam, interview with the author, New Delhi. The representation of economic growth in terms of the GDP is not unique to Kalam. In the years following the economic reforms that were launched in 1991, the GDP became the object of intense fascination within Indian elite circles and media spheres. A high GDP was seen as a demonstration of the success of the reforms, especially when compared with the infamous "Hindu rate of growth," an expression used to mock the low economic growth (3 to 4 percent on average) of the decades preceding the reforms.

10. In *The Economization of Life*, Michelle Murphy argues that although everyone agrees that GDP, as a single number, necessarily misrepresents the complexity of economic life. Yet an index like the GDP carries affective stimulus in surplus of any rational principle: As a felt reality, a measure such as the GDP, Murphy suggests, carries intensities and potentialities in excess of quantification and the many social forms it is taking: "Economy is capitalism's secular divine and GDP its oracle. It demands faith even if on earth its worldly manifestations come in the form of blight and hype. What won't we go for GDP?" (Murphy 2017, 25). It should be noted, however, that Kalam himself promoted the adoption of a National Prosperity Index (NPI) that would combine GDP with the measure of the reduction of people living Below the Poverty Line (BPL) and a measure of social values. Kalam's concern was that GDP was not reflected in the quality of life of a large number of people, especially the poorest.

11. Anna Greenspan sums up the project in these terms: "The project of branding India works by reconceptualizing those things which are stereotypically Indian in such a way as to show that, no matter how ancient, they were always closely intermeshed with the digital technology of today" (Greenspan 2004, 142). Chopra rather insists on the Hindu nationalist version of the narrative: "An insistence on the universalism and globality of Hinduism, a focus on the inherent scientificity of Hindu ethos and culture and the technological expertise of Hindus, ambivalence toward the shifting signifier of the 'West,' an essentialized interpretation of Hindu and Indian identity accompanied by antiminority prejudice, a rejection of Left ideologies, an embrace of free market and capitalism, and a rejection of Indian secularism" (Chopra 2008, 8–9).

12. Kalam (2003, 38) writes, "Ancient India was a knowledge society and a leader in many intellectual pursuits, particularly in the fields of mathematics, medicine and astron-

omy. A renaissance is imperative for us to once again become a knowledge superpower rather than simply providing cheap labor in areas of high technology."

13. As was noted by Mamadou Diouf, we can find a similar rehabilitation in the work of the Senegalese historian and anthropologist Cheikh Anta Diop, who argued that Africa had a rich cultural and scientific heritage that had been suppressed and distorted by colonialism and racism. Just like Indian intellectuals and nationalists, Cheikh Anta Diop rejected colonial knowledge that "assigns to India as well as to Africa a passivity that radically withdraws them from any possibility of change and considers them as resistant to historical transformations" (Diouf 1999, 9; translation mine).

14. To participate in the Pan-African e-Network, Indian hospitals had to be selected as part of tender process. All of the leading hospital chains in the country responded to the call. Out of the twelve tertiary care hospitals selected, nine were private hospitals, generally part of corporate chains. Three public hospitals, among the country's leading medical institutes, were also connected.

15. Interview with the author, Bangalore.

16. For example, see this article in *Wired* magazine reporting on the "Indian superbug" from the annual Interscience Conference on Antimicrobial Agents and Chemotherapy in September 2010: "In South Asia, several of the researchers pointed out, antibiotic overuse is common, diarrheal disease is endemic, and municipal sanitation is available to only about half of the more than 1 billion population. That's practically a recipe for the rapid spread of genetic material carried by gut bacteria—and the economic realities of the subcontinent make it unlikely that any of those conditions are going to be remedied soon" (McKenna 2010).

17. Interestingly, however, while the Indian government rejected the paper, the controversy nevertheless led to the launch of a committee to frame a policy for antibiotic use, and control and mapping of hospital-acquired infections.

18. A rapid search using the Factiva database for newspaper articles, for example, turns up 827 publications that mention the Pan-African e-Network, including 677 in India.

19. According to the Skoch Renaissance Award website, the award is "conferred on corporate organisations which demonstrate outstanding leadership through sustainable practices and sensible corporate social responsibilities. . . . The Skoch Renaissance Award considers corporate entities that have contributed significantly to India's growth through an exemplary, sustainable & balanced business performance." See https://award.skoch.in for a list of past awardees.

20. *Connecting Hearts: India's Pan African e-Network* was released in 2011. It is available here: https://www.youtube.com/watch?v=73LMVBnPacg.

21. *Connecting Hearts & Minds: India's PAN Africa Story* was released in 2012. It is available here: https://www.youtube.com/watch?v=eBUmdnab9io. Another, longer version is available in (very poorly translated) French: https://www.youtube.com/watch?v=KFj6WQgXJ60.

22. To the best of my knowledge, *Bridging the Gap* was never released online. It was displayed during exhibitions and conferences. I was handed a French version of the film.

23. Pranab Mukherjee, who inaugurated the pilot project in 2007, and then PAN itself on February 26, 2009, later succeeded Abdul Kalam as the thirteenth president of India—a position he occupied between July 2012 and July 2017 (the very month that the network ceased its activities). Just like Kalam's, Mukherjee's political trajectory was therefore very much intertwined with PAN. While Kalam was nominated by the Hindu nationalist BJP, Mukherjee was a member of the Indian National Congress. However, just like Kalam, the glorious heritage of ancient India (including the philosophy of vasudhaiva kutumbakam) was key to his brand of nationalism. Largely because of this, Mukherjee and Kalam both

shared the rare capacity to attract cross-party support, which contributed in their acceptability as presidents.

24. This is what Kaur and Blom Hansen refer to as an "aesthetic of arrival" (Kaur and Blom Hansen 2016). Think of Dr. Prathap Reddy, in the opening scene of this chapter: the global expansion of the Indian health care industry, of which he is a spearhead, was raising India on the "top of the world."

25. As was recently noted by Venkatachalam and Banik (2022), this notion runs through the recent history of India-Africa cooperation, and it was already entrenched in Bandung. Abdul Kalam instead generally uses the notion of *jagadguru*, a Sanskrit notion which translates as "guru of the universe" or "world leader" (Kalam 2003, 76).

26. A scene in *Connecting Hearts* tells the story of a telemedicine encounter in which a chronically ill patient was cured using the network. Images of the patient sitting beside the treating doctor in Senegal are displayed. Hence I was surprised when, watching the film, I recognized the patient as a Senegalese IT technician working on other telemedicine projects at CHNU Fann in Dakar. When I mentioned this to the "patient-technician" and his colleagues over lunch, we had a good time laughing.

27. For work that examines global forms of medical experimentation and knowledge production in Africa, see Geissler et al. 2008; Nguyen 2010; Mkhwanazi 2020; Peterson et al. 2015; and Rottenburg 2009.

28. See Adams 2016 as well as Kelly and McGoey 2018.

29. Drawing on the writings of Pignarre and Stengers (2011) on the magical temper of capitalism, Adrian Mackenzie underlines the distinction between validation and verification as being critical to wireless development projects. The emphasis on validation, I believe, applies to the Pan-African e-Network: "The key term here is verification. This is a contentious statement from the perspective of, say, an econometrician, but in terms of pragmatism, understood as a technique for the construction of ideas, capitalism does not verify, it only validates. Verification is an eminently practical procedure interested in consequences. It might entail experiments, tracking of consequences, and orientation toward further actions. Validation is anti-pragmatic in that it seeks to assert something and hold the assumption in place. It is resistant to overflow and overabundance" (Mackenzie 2010, 173).

30. Our focus on the speculative logic of PAN, on what it *does*, is inspired by Bruno Latour's refusal to demote critique to a mere question debunking hype, discourse, or dreams. Latour writes, "The fairy position is very well known and is used over and over again by many social scientists who associate criticism with antifetishism. The role of the critic is then to show that what the naïve believers are doing with objects is simply a projection of their wishes onto a material entity that does nothing at all by itself. Here they have diverted to their petty use the prophetic fulmination against idols 'they have mouths and speak not, they have ears and hear not,' but they use this prophecy to decry the very objects of belief—gods, fashion, poetry, sport, desire, you name it—to which naïve believers cling with so much intensity" (Latour 2004, 237–38).

31. Sunder Rajan refers to Marx's allusion to the "theological" character of commodity: to its mystical and magical nature by which it can operate abstraction and become the mediator of social bonds (Sunder Rajan 2006, 18).

32. Significant contribution to the "new materialist" turn include Barad 2007; Bennett 2010; Braun and Whatmore 2010; Connolly 2011; Coole and Frost 2010; Ingold 2011; Jackson 2018; Latour 1993; and Massumi 2002. More recently, tenants of object-oriented ontology (OOO) have pushed things further, making an argument for the independent existence of things and their capacity to relate to human beings in ways not mediated by human consciousness or intentionality. OOO insists on the opaque and nonrelational aspects of material entities and how they present themselves to thought in their own right.

For a summary, see Bryant, Srnicek, and Harman 2011 as well as Harman 2018. For an instructive debate between Graham Harman and Bruno Latour on the topic, see Latour, Harman, and Erdélyi 2011.

33. I paraphrase here from Lauren Berlant (2011, 30) on the aesthetic autonomy of a poem.

34. I borrow here from Webb Keane's comment on Joshua Barker's study of the satellite discourse and the political meaning of the satellite in Indonesia. See the full comment at the end of Barker (2005).

35. This is obviously only one example of the mutually constitutive relation between economic interest and the enjoyment of spectacular political promises. William Mazzarella provides us with an example of desires being animated by a radically different although contemporary spatial form: "One might think that Trump's endlessly repeated promise to build a border wall between the United States and Mexico reaped an ill wind of anti-immigrant sentiment. And one would be right. But one would also have to acknowledge that the wall embodies a spectacular and grandiose promise of enjoyment, far beyond whatever function it might have as a physical barrier" (Mazzarella 2019, 120).

36. To borrow Geoffrey Bowker's description of globalization, the satellite form seeks to "impose a uniform representational time and space on a heterogenous collection of lived spaces and histories" (Bowker 1995, 55).

37. Similarly, the works of Harold Innis and Buckminster Fuller, along with McLuhan's writings on the "global village," have all insisted on the patterns of expansion and unification afforded by satellite connectivity.

38. As was famously argued by Gilbert Simondon in his critique of the hylomorphic model, form is neither abstract nor imposed upon raw materials: The relation between matter and form is not made between inert matter and form coming from the outside (*dehors*). The operation by which an object having form and matter emerges, suggests Simondon, can't be represented by the matter-form couple. What the form-matter couple inevitably misses is a complicated series of energetic exchanges that mediate between matter and form—for instance, between clay and mold in the case of brick-forming, examined in detail by Simondon. What is neglected is the ongoing process of formation, the "pre-individual" in which "form, matter, and energy preexist in the system" (Simondon 1989, 16; translation is mine).

39. In *Speaking into the Air*, Peters argues that the concept of communication as we know it originates from a "spiritualist tradition" that he traces back to Saint Augustine, British empiricism, and nineteenth-century spiritualism, where it took its current shape. Spiritualism, suggests Peters, "foreshadows modern communications and the problem of how to conjure the credible presence of an absent body for an audience remote in time, space, or degree" (Peters 1999, 71). This problem of presence was also accompanied by the practical and philosophical problem of remote action, of operations that work at a distance, without touch. "In the seventeenth century," writes Peters, "the term was consistently used to refer to what the Scholastics called *actio in distans*—action at a distance. Since at least the Scholastics, action at a distance has been a problem in natural philosophy: How can one body influence another without palpably touching it?" (Peters 1999, 78).

40. In *Marvelous Clouds*, Peters develops an environmental view of media in which he presents the *medium*—singular of media—as the missing link, stepping in to "fill the environmental gaps" to explain action or contact at a distance. Medium, like its sibling milieu, is the intermediate agent in the transmission of entities and specifically of human signals and meanings (Peters 2015, 46–49).

41. As Mazzarella also notes, Marcel Mauss thus describes magical action: "Distance does not preclude contact. Desires and images can be immediately realized" (Mazzarella 2017, 37).

42. Here is Kalam on national unity: "What we need today is a vision for the nation which can bring unity. It is when we accept India in all its splendid glory that, with a shared past as a base, we can look forward to a shared future of peace and prosperity, of creation and abundance. Our past is there with us forever. It has to be nurtured in good faith, not destroyed in exercises of political one-upmanship. The developed India will not be a nation of cities. It will be a network of prosperous villages empowered by telemedicine, tele-education and e-commerce" (Kalam 2003, 116).

43. This is a fictitious name. I also do not mention the hospital either, for confidentiality reasons.

44. Being admitted to one of the 16 IITs is no small feat. In 2012, 512,000 applicants participated in the IITs' joint entrance examination. Of these, 9,647 students were accepted into one of the institutions, which is less than 2 percent.

45. The Indian IT industry had been growing very quickly, more or less doubling in size, in the years preceding PAN. For discussions of living and working conditions in the Indian IT sector around the years PAN was launched, see Biao 2007; Fuller and Narasimhan 2007; and Nisbett 2009.

46. On "waiting" or "time passing" as a strategic response to underemployment in India, especially among educated lower-middle-class young men just like Krishnan, see Jeffrey 2010.

47. Interview with the author, New Delhi. An Indian entrepreneur similarly complained about the difficulty of finding qualified workers willing to expatriate themselves to Africa: "In India, it is difficult to get people to go to Africa. Lots of Indians are vegetarians. Lots of Indians are very scared of this whole idea about Africa. So it's a very intriguing thing if you look at it" (interview with the author, Bangalore).

48. These vacations had an impact on the smooth running of PAN's activities. The absence of engineers could put teleconsultations of CME sessions on hold, especially in locations with only one PAN engineer.

49. A summary of the coin collection and of the awards received can be found in Mullick (2017) as well as on the website of Guinness World Records: https://www.guinness worldrecords.com/world-records/387431-largest-collection-of-bi-metallic-coins.

50. Underlying this notion of the "waiting room" is a developmentalist and indeed teleological conception of history. In practice, however, the totalizing thrusts of history are always modified and interrupted. On this topic, see Dipesh Chakrabarty's discussion of a Heideggerian relationship to the future in the epilogue to *Provincializing Europe*. Put roughly, Charkabarty insists that historicism and totalizing conceptions of reason shall always be put in tension with other ways of being in the world (Chakrabarty 2000). The future that "will be," Chakrabarty suggests, never completely swamps the many incomplete, inchoate futures that already are (254).

51. It is not my aim to provide an overview of the extremely prolific anthropological literature on the gift. However, essential work includes Godbout and Caille 1998; Godelier 1999; Graeber 2001; Gregory 2015; Sahlins [2017] 1972; Strathern 1988; and Weiner 1992. For a recent summary of the anthropological discussions of gift exchange, see Yan 2023. In French, the publications of the Revue du MAUSS (Mouvement anti-utilitariste dans les sciences sociales) are unavoidable. See https://www.cairn.info/revue-du-mauss1 .htm. For discussions of gift giving in global health contexts, see Kenworthy 2014 and Minn 2022.

52. In a comment on Sprenger's paper, Pickles picks his side: "For instance, Sprenger writes that because gifts do not determine a return but rather create an expectation, the gift 'opens up future possibilities.' This is not so; expectation narrows the field of possibility, even if it doesn't do so to quite the same extent as obligation would" (Pickles 2023, 95–96). I remain more ambivalent.

5. MAPS AND TERRITORIES

1. According to Banik, Venkatachalam, and Modi (2023, 10), a total of 6,771 CME sessions were held between 2009 and 2017.

2. During my stay at CHNU Fann, there was only one morning when doctors showed up to attend a session in neurology, titled "Clinical Approach to Dementia." Then, one more doctor came for the next session on "Medical Aspects of Kidney Transplant." Interestingly, none of these doctors were from CHNU Fann. They had come from the Hôpital Aristide Le Dantec and the Hôpital Principal de Dakar, two neighboring public hospitals. Mostly medical residents, they had recently heard about PAN and came out of curiosity. At the end of the session, they asked the engineers about the possibility of having CME sessions in French. Jean-Louis later explained to me that sometimes TCIL hired a translator to translate sessions into French, but only from the Dr. Balabha Nanavati Hospital in Mumbai. The translator did simultaneous translation and introduced the slides displayed in French. Jean-Louis specified, however, that she made many mistakes in the translation of medical terms. On two occasions, he intervened with Dr. Balabha Nanavati Hospital to stop the translation because the doctors preferred to listen to the session in English rather than in poor French. I have never myself witnessed such a translated session.

3. Speakers received financial compensation for their participation in PAN. While a teleconsultation paid between INR1,000 and INR1,500 per hour, the fee for a CME session is INR5,000, or just over US$60. The choice of topic for the session was always at the discretion of the speaker.

4. There are technical reasons for this. Put roughly, the windows on the screen the lecturer was looking at could not be changed. From the control room, the engineer and I could see other audiences. But the speaker could see only the same audience from the beginning to the end of the presentation—which could lead to all sorts of awkward situations, including witnessing rooms that had emptied themselves of the few people attending or people sitting there without paying much attention.

5. To try to compensate for this unfortunate situation, engineers in an Indian hospital could at times ask a colleague in Africa to sit in one of the chairs as if he or she were attending the session. During my stay at Fann, I indeed witnessed this happening. Although engineers at Fann did not approve of the strategy, they sometimes complied since they acknowledged that giving a lecture that no one was attending could be demoralizing.

6. Interview with the author, Chennai.

7. Interview with the author, Chennai.

8. Sandra Calkins makes a similar argument about the literature on infrastructure in the Global South with stories that paint a "heroic picture of tinkering and improvisation": "It is undeniably important to highlight the creativity and agency of people who, lacking resources, have to make do and stitch fraying infrastructures together. This holds true especially in African settings, where people still are far too often portrayed as largely victims of world historical processes. . . . And yet, at times this important correction of ways of writing about Africa has fed its opposite—a romance of improvisation, of repair, recycling and reuse that backgrounds the darker side, the humiliation and the dangers that can also be lurking when people step into infrastructural gaps" (Calkins 2021, 708).

9. This is also the response that Mkhwanazi (2020) gives to her own question in a different paper published a few years later about Soka Uncobe, the same failed medical circumcision campaign implemented in eSwatini. While there are many similarities in the implementation of Soka Uncobe and PAN, and the factors explaining their poor uptake are often alike, a key difference lies in the fact that Soka Uncobe was largely undermined by the obsession with numbers and the centrality of quantification practices that has become dominant in global health. In PAN, in contrast, there was no such practices. Control in PAN was not a matter of calculation but rather of topology and spatial ordering.

10. I approach digital networks as both idea and thing, which compromises any easy distinction between the theoretical and the empirical. In doing so, I am inspired by the work of media scholars including Wendy Hui Kyong Chun (Chun and Cotte 2020; Chun 2015); Anna Munster (2013); Alexander Galloway and Eugene Thacker (2007); Adrian Mackenzie (2010); Steven Shaviro (2003); Tung-Hui Hu (2015); and John Durham Peters (2015), among many others.

11. Interview with the author, New Delhi.

12. Interview with the author, Chennai.

13. Interview with the author, New Delhi.

14. Interview with the author, New Delhi.

15. Each country connected to PAN selected a local coordinator for the project, usually affiliated with the Ministry of Telecommunications. The coordinator was also in charge of identifying the hospital that would be connected to PAN.

16. Interview with the author, Dakar.

17. Interview with the author, Addis Ababa.

18. Interview with the author, Dakar.

19. Interview with the author, New Delhi.

20. The issue of resistance to change is not unique to PAN and is widely recognized as a major obstacle to the uptake of telemedicine. As a recent review of literature suggested, "Telemedicine requires significant changes to the existing workflows and many staff and providers have to invest time in training new workflows and techniques, and this affects both efficiency and effectiveness of the care" (Scott Kruse et al. 2018, 8). User resistance has been documented worldwide. For extensive discussions, see Mair et al. 2007; Brewster et al. 2014; and Xue et al. 2015.

21. Interview with the author, Addis Ababa.

22. This stands in contrast to the rhetorics of "natural relationships" between India and Africa that PAN promised to materialize. Or, rather, it emphasizes the teleological vision of development embedded in resurgent India-Africa cooperation. As Indian stakeholders often explained to me, India was particularly well suited to provide such expertise to Africa because it was, until recently, in a similar position (that is, of underdevelopment).

23. Interview with the author, Dakar.

24. Interview with author. Although Senegalese doctors who used the network had a good command of written English, many mentioned struggles with the accent of Indian doctors, especially when they spoke rapidly.

25. Engineers on the PAN sites where I spent the most time were aware that French was my mother tongue and that I could help to do such routine translation. I was required to do this only on a few occasions, however.

26. Interview with the author.

27. Interview with the author.

28. In their study of the implementation of PAN at the Komfo Anokye Teaching Hospital in Ghana, Afarikumah and Kwankam also note that scheduling was a key factor explaining poor attendance at CME sessions. A doctor thus summarized the situation: "It is normally around 11 to 12 and that was like the middle of the day and for us if you are in our primary care, we are given slots so you would have to be in a clinic from 8 a.m. to 2 p.m. So you can't just go and listen and then stay there for one hour. It's not the best for Komfo Anokye so I used to attend when I didn't have the clinic but sometimes you really want to listen and you have a clinic so you are torn between the two. The timing was the problem. So, my recommendation is that if it was early in the morning or in the middle that would maybe help a larger number of people to attend" (Afarikumah and Kwankam 2013, 81). Another study, conducted after PAN's activities were over, also noted that scheduling conflicts were an issue for CME attendance in Ghana (Banik, Venkatachalam, and Modi 2023).

29. This was also noted by Bénédicte Bazin in her master's thesis, which was largely dedicated to the project. Bazin noted how, according to a consultant working for the Ministry of Health of Senegal, the poor utilization of PAN was similar to having "a Ferrari in the garage" (Bazin 2019, 62). Bazin notes that even though most clinicians at CHNU Fann tended to appreciate the network, the imposition of the schedule was a major obstacle to its utilization.

30. Interview with the author.

31. Drawing from fieldwork carried out in Mozambique, De Bruyn (2018) also notes that PAN's top-down turnkey approach was a decisive factor in its poor local uptake: "In conclusion, the top-down, standalone and blueprint approach limits the agency and appropriation of the project by its end users as well as an effective transfer of Indian expertise to other contexts" (De Bruyn 2018, 14).

32. A PAN engineer in charge of the project in one of the participating Indian hospitals noted, "The problem is the personal contact. We cannot communicate directly with them. Only through TCIL we can communicate. . . . But unless we talk to the local people, like we usually do with our other telemedicine networks, we cannot know what are their expectations, what is the problem there. That's another drawback. In Africa, we don't know who to contact! If we go through TCIL, the process is complicated. TCIL are working fine, but there are many levels. Many forces are there. It's difficult to make things move quickly" (interview with the author).

33. For advocates of an emergent change approach, change is not "a series of linear events within a given period of time" but rather a "continuous, open-ended process of adaptation to changing circumstances and conditions" (By 2005, 375). Emergent change is particularly suited to deal with environments with high uncertainty levels. For papers providing a fine overview of emergent change theory, see Bamford and Forrester 2003 and Burnes 2004.

34. Afarikumah and Kwankam also conclude that the architecture of the network, and the hub-and-spoke topology in particular, severely limited the power of PAN: "While the project aimed at providing Internet connectivity to African institutions, the architecture limited these institutions to connecting to Indian centers only. It was not an interconnected network of African institutions but a system of African institutions all connected to Indian centers, but not otherwise linked to one another. . . . Experience showed that sharing of experiences and knowledge among the nodes was very limited. Thus, Nigeria and Ghana, which conceivably have a lot in common in terms of medical education challenges, could not share experiences directly through the eNetwork. The architecture thus constrained the network to focusing on those medical education challenges where the solutions could be found in the Indian centers" (Afarikumah and Kwankam 2013, 82).

35. Banik, Venkatachalam, and Modi (2023, 18) also note that PAN stakeholders in India, "including the implementing agency and project partners, did not pay adequate attention to how Indian expertise could be best tailored to address the needs of the host hospitals on the African continent." They further explain, "[PAN] was meant to be an Africa-wide programme, but diverse economic and social landscapes characterise the continent, and a one-size-fits-all approach will not work" (22).

36. Drawing from the study of an electronic patient record (EPR) system in Denmark, Casper Bruun Jensen (2006) suggests that such a "technologic" of project implementation takes root in the separation of the technical from the organizational domain, which locates them in different ontological and analytical domains. As it is blind to the entanglements, in practice, of the technical and the organizational, this dichotomous conception tends to lead to a prioritization of technical expansion over the organizational dimension of project implementation. For instance, Jensen suggests that it contributes to a systematic underestimation of the capacity of health care practices to change the outcomes of EPR implementation efforts. This affects the way projects' successes and failures are analyzed,

as technology tends to be perceived as neutral and an extra component—"something intangibly 'social' or 'cultural' or 'organisational'" (Jensen 2006, 43)—is identified as the source of resistance to efficient adoption.

37. A paper published in 2020 in *Lancet Digital Health* thus summarized the growing scientific consensus within the literature: "To make digital health flourish within sub-Saharan Africa, enabling environments need to be created that are firmly anchored within the local context, driven by African needs, endorsed by decision makers such as national governments and supported by global key players such as the United Nations and WHO" (Holst et al. 2020, e161).

38. Another sign of this divide lies in the simple fact that although the project had a strong health component, the ministries of health of participating countries were not involved. Rather, officials from ministries of telecommunications or information technology were generally elected to oversee PAN's activities in collaboration with TCIL. The same was true in India, as TCIL (an engineering and technology company) and the Ministry of External Affairs were in charge of the project. The Ministry of Health and Family Welfare of India was thus not involved at all in the project.

39. Seminal work along these lines includes Akrich (1992); Barad (2007); Mol (2002); and Pickering (1995), among many others.

40. On that matter, Woolgar and Lezaun (2013, 324) write, "Objects do not acquire a particular meaning in, or because of, a given context; they cannot be accounted for by reference to the external circumstances of their existence. Rather, objects are brought into being, they are realised in the course of a certain practical activity, and when that happens, they crystallise, provisionally, a particular reality, they invoke the temporary action of a set of circumstances."

41. Afarikumah and Kwankam (2013, 82) make a similar observation about PAN in Ghana: "The staff perceives the project an as optional system. Technically, the staff consider the system as an IT device and thus, are focused more on maintaining the mainstream IT equipment."

42. With PAN, India had to do something original, the ISRO scientist recalled. The country had to distinguish itself, to find a way to do something that would bring to the forefront its expertise in cutting-edge fields and benefit the masses: "You have to do something that no others do. Something different. Which really benefits the population" (interview with the author).

43. Scaling up, Bruno Latour (2007a, 141) also reminds us, "is a tough, surprising adventure filled with twists and detours."

44. I am here inspired by Hannah Appel's call to pay attention to what she calls the "licit life of capitalism"—namely, to practices that have become legally sanctioned or widely adopted, even as they are contested or failing. Appel writes, "This attention to the licit undertakes an anthropology of capitalism that proceeds not (or not only) from a sociology of error but from the question of how what currently exists has been stabilized (Roitman 2014, 78; see also de Goede 2005). Rather than only a (mis)representation to be deconstructed, capitalism is a constant construction project to be traced through research" (Appel 2019, 22).

45. An Indian neurosurgeon and frequent user of PAN suggested to me, "I have spent most of my life working in a public hospital. So I have tasted both. I know what a corporate hospital is, what is international medicine, but I know the realities of the world. Most tele-consultants here are all American Board certified, or Canadian or English. They went abroad, spent 10 years, 15 years and then came back. They're out of touch with reality. I've been to Africa, I've visited several hospitals and according to me, Africa is what India was in 1980! Or 1975. So they ask us for a consultation, my oncologist says: 'Get a PET CT done.' But there's no PET CT in the whole bloody country! You understand? So our doctors also are to blame. I just go back to what I used to do 20 years ago and that's it."

46. Adams, Murphy, and Clarke thus comment on how development logics can make places appear "backward in time": "Promissory capital speculation and development logics render some places as backward in time, needing anticipatory investment, while other places are deemed already at the cusp of the 'new' future, marked by the virtue of rapid change. This goes unquestioned because speculative capital operates as if the virtues of movement into valued futures are already known. Promissory market logics not only find new sites of investment, but produce them as problematized domains" (Adams, Murphy, and Clarke 2009, 251).

47. Whether real or imagined, distance, note Sud and Sánchez-Ancochea, "reinforces otherness and justifies typecasting" (2022, 1128). This certainly applies to PAN.

48. Again James Scott is useful here. In his work on everyday resistance, Scott has argued that passive resistance can be just as effective as more overt forms of resistance in undermining the power of state authorities and development projects. Everyday forms of resistance may include foot dragging, escape, sarcasm, passivity, laziness, repeated misunderstandings, disloyalty, avoidance, or theft. Distance, for Scott, plays a key role in the ability of people to resist state control. For Scott, the physical distance of rural communities from centers of power, along with the friction of terrain, can make it difficult for state authorities to exert control over these communities. See, for example, Scott 1985.

49. Glissant defines opacity as a diversity that exceeds categories of identifiable difference. Opacity is not a natural quality but a mode of active resistance that emerges in response to particular political problems. For Glissant, the right to opacity appears as an ethical stance against imperial conquest and domination. By insisting that the West is a project, not a place, Glissant situates opacity in opposition to the Enlightenment project of knowledge that valued universal models and categories: a project that worked through a process of understanding dependent on operations of reduction and hierarchization. To assert one's right to opacity is to refuse to be known only on the terms of the colonizer and for the benefit of the colonizer. Opacity does not appear as an antirational mode of thinking but rather as resistance to the light of (Western) understanding to preserve diversity and advance nonhierarchical exchange. Opacity is an unknowability—and therefore a poetics, for Glissant—that constitutes the world. And it must be defended if any radically democratic project is to succeed.

50. As was noted by philosopher Sylvia Wynters in a fine discussion of Glissant, disruption above all referred to "the premise of an acultural and absolute model of the human" (Wynter 1989, 645).

51. Around the time PAN was launched, there already was momentum for telemedicine in Senegal. Several projects had been launched in previous years, including at CHNU Fann but also in other public and district health centers. While most of these projects ended in their early stages, research carried out by Ly et al. (2017) shows that the attitude of health professionals in Senegal was more positive than negative toward telemedicine and that most were likely to use it in their professional activities.

52. Poet, cultural theorist, and Senegal's first president, Léopold Sédar Senghor promoted the notion of the "Civilisation of the Universal," which posits that all cultures and civilizations have a unique contribution to universal values and global community. This idea is a central tenet of Senghor's Négritude philosophy, which emphasizes the role of African cultural identity in shaping a universal civilization. The Civilisation of the Universal is "a symbiosis of the different civilisations," shaped by the "encounter of giving and receiving" (Senghor 1998, 447). Glissant argued for a more dynamic and flexible concept of identity that recognizes the constant evolution and movement of cultures.

53. I am not suggesting that PAN was disseminated from a center to peripheries but rather that the network contributed to *making* these new geographies. For a discussion, see Harvey, Jensen, and Morita 2016.

EPILOGUE

1. Interview with the author, Bangalore.

2. Funding, noted an Africa Union report dedicated to PAN, was the main challenge (African Union 2018). After eight years of activities, the question had become: Who is going to fund the network's operations?

3. Email correspondence with the author.

4. In practice, however, only 3 percent of all COVID-19 vaccine doses delivered in 2021 went to Africa, although it represents one-fifth of the global population (WHO 2023). John Nkengasong, the head of the Africa Centres for Disease Control, considered that Africa was let down by the Serum Institute of India, the world's biggest vaccine maker (Al Jazeera News Agency 2021). In March 2021, as millions of doses made by the Serum Institute of India of the AstraZeneca vaccine were bound for Africa, India indeed issued a ban on the export of the vaccine, contributing to a supply gap when African countries needed the vaccine the most. More recently, the publication of vaccine contracts between South Africa and vaccine providers revealed that the country greatly overpaid for the procurement of vaccines and that "the biggest apparent markup paid by South Africa was to the Serum Institute of India, maker of the Oxford AstraZeneca vaccine" (Dyer 2023). Again, then, the great moral claims and political spectacle of "vaccine diplomacy" did not necessarily sit well with India's actual engagement, which showed signs of the same brand of vaccine nationalism, stockpiling, and profit seeking as other major vaccine producers.

5. Gandhi, Dilip Menon suggests in a comment on the #GandhiMustFall movement, "is a metaphor for the Indian presence in Africa and histories of both Indian racism as well as commercial wealth." Menon notes the irony, however, of Gandhi standing in for Indian presence in Africa at this particular juncture in Indian politics: "The irony is that, while Gandhi becomes increasingly sidelined in the maelstrom of Indian politics, in Africa he has come to stand in for the Indian presence" (Menon 2017).

6. On COVID-19 as a vector for Hindu nationalism in India, see Subramaniam 2021. India is obviously not the only country where such a parochial turn was taken in recent years. In the wake of COVID-19, nationalist revivals across the globe increasingly blur the line between care and containment, exposure and enclosure.

7. It is noteworthy that Arogya Bharti is also the name of a nongovernmental organization in India that promotes health and well-being, with close ties to the Rashtriya Swayamsevak Sangh (RSS), a Hindu nationalist organization (that happened to play a critical role in shaping Prime Minister Modi's political career).

8. In 2016, Rajiv Bhatia, former Indian ambassador and director general of the Indian Council of World Affairs, suggested that Modi's foreign policy mirrored a continued belief in the soft power of vasudhaiva kutumbakam but also some of the key "hard power" teachings of the Arthashastra, the ancient Indian manual of great-power diplomacy and international statecraft. India's ambition to become a major power, according to Bhatia, reflects the impulse to be an ideal universal leader—a *chakravartin*, in Arthashastra. *Vasudhaiva kutumbakam* and *Arthashastra*, in such instances, refer not only to the proper conduct of government but also to a civilizational legacy and values that shall model India's engagement in the world (Bhatia 2016).

References

Abraham, Itty. 1996. "Science and Power in the Postcolonial State." *Alternatives: Global, Local, Political* 21 (3): 321–39. https://doi.org/10.1177/030437549602100303.

Abraham, Itty. 2007. "The Future of Indian Foreign Policy." *Economic and Political Weekly* 42 (42): 4209–12. https://www.jstor.org/stable/40276567.

Abraham, Itty. 2014. *How India Became Territorial: Foreign Policy, Diaspora, Geopolitics.* Stanford, CA: Stanford University Press.

Acharya, Mahapragya, and A. P. J. Abdul Kalam. 2009. *The Family and the Nation.* New Delhi, India: HarperCollins.

Adams, Vincanne, ed. 2016. *Metrics: What Counts in Global Health.* Durham, NC: Duke University Press.

Adams, Vincanne, Dominique Behague, Carlo Caduff, Ilana Löwy, and Francisco Ortega. 2019. "Re-imagining Global Health through Social Medicine." *Global Public Health* 14 (10): 1–18. https://doi.org/10.1080/17441692.2019.1587639.

Adams, Vincanne, Michelle Murphy, and Adele E. Clarke. 2009. "Anticipation: Technoscience, Life, Affect, Temporality." *Subjectivity* 28 (1): 246–65. https://doi.org/10.1057/sub.2009.18.

Adibe, Jideofor. 2017. "Impact of Xenophobic Attacks against Africans in India on Afro-India Relations." *Journal of African Foreign Affairs* 4 (1–2): 85–97. https://hdl.handle.net/10520/EJC-8b3491c0a.

Afarikumah, Eben, and S. Yunkap Kwankam. 2013. "Deploying Actor-Network Theory to Analyse Telemedicine Implementation in Ghana." *Science Journal of Public Health* 1 (2): 77–84. https://doi.org/10.11648/j.sjph.20130102.15.

African Union. 2018. "First Progress Report of the Chairperson of the Commission on the Pan African e-Network on Tele-education and Tele-Medicine." Last modified March 29. 2018. http://www.peaceau.org/uploads/auc.report.panafrican.e-network.prc.29.03.18.pdf.

Agathangelou, Anna M. 2016. "Casting Off the 'Heavenly Rule Book': Bandung's Poetic Revolutionary Solidarities." In *Meanings of Bandung: Postcolonial Orders and Decolonial Visions*, edited by Quỳnh N. Phạm and Robbie Shilliam, 101–12. London: Rowman & Littlefield.

Akrich, Madeleine. 1992. "The De-scription of Technical Objects." In *Shaping Technology/Building Society*, edited by Wiebe E. Bijker and John Law, 205–24. Cambridge, MA: MIT Press.

Al Dahdah, Marine. 2017. "Health at Her Fingertips: Development, Gender and Empowering Mobile Technologies." *Gender, Technology and Development* 21 (1–2): 135–51. https://doi.org/10.1080/09718524.2017.1385701.

Al Dahdah, Marine. 2019. "From Evidence-Based to Market-Based mHealth: Itinerary of a Mobile (for) Development Project." *Science, Technology, & Human Values* 44 (6): 1048–67. https://doi.org/10.1177/0162243918824657.

Al Jazeera News Agency. 2021. "India's Serum Institute Let Africa Down on Vaccines: Africa CDC." *Al Jazeera.* Last modified December 9, 2021. https://www.aljazeera.com/news/2021/12/9/indias-serum-institute-let-africa-down-on-vaccines-africa-cdc.

Anderson, Warwick. 2014. "Making Global Health History: The Postcolonial Worldli-
ness of Biomedicine." *Social History of Medicine* 27 (2): 372–84. https://doi.org
/10.1093/shm/hkt126.

Aneja, Urvashi. 2015. "India-Africa Summit: Is It Possible for One Country to Share a
Vision with an Entire Continent?" Last modified October 28, 2015. https://scroll
.in/article/765026/india-africa-summit-is-it-possible-for-one-country-to-share
-a-vision-with-an-entire-continent.

ANI. 2018. "PM Modi invokes 'Vasudhaiva Kutumbakam' at World Economic Forum."
Business Standard, January 23. https://www.business-standard.com/article/news
-ani/pm-modi-invokes-vasudhaiva-kutumbakam-at-world-economic-forum-11
8012300901_1.html.

Appel, Hannah. 2019. *The Licit Life of Capitalism: US Oil in Equatorial Guinea.* Durham,
NC: Duke University Press.

Appel, Hannah, Nikhil Anand, and Akhil Gupta. 2018. "Introduction: Temporality, Politics, and the Promise of Infrastructure." In *The Promise of Infrastructure*, edited by
Nikhil Anand, Akhil Gupta, and Hannah Appel, 1–38. Durham, NC: Duke University Press.

Aranda-Jan, Clara B., Neo Mohutsiwa-Dibe, and Svetla Loukanova. 2014. "Systematic
Review on What Works, What Does Not Work and Why of Implementation of
Mobile Health (mHealth) Projects in Africa." *BMC Public Health* 14: 188. https://
doi.org/10.1186/1471-2458-14-188.

Arbab, Farah. 2006. "India's Growing Ties with Africa." *Strategic Studies* 26, no. 4 (Winter 2006): 33–60. https://jstor.org/stable/45242367.

Arnold, David. 1993. *Colonizing the Body: State Medicine and Epidemic Disease in Nineteenth-Century India.* Berkeley: University of California Press.

Arnold, David. 2013. "Nehruvian Science and Postcolonial India." *Isis* 104 (2): 360–70.
https://doi.org/10.1086/670954.

Aronson, Sidney H. 1977. "The Lancet on the Telephone 1876–1975." *Medical History*
21 (1): 69–87. https://doi.org/10.1017/S0025727300037182.

Babu, Gireesh. 2014. "Apollo Hospitals to Expand Operations in African Countries."
Business Standard, February 9. https://www.business-standard.com/article/com
panies/apollo-hospitals-to-expand-operations-in-african-countries-114020900
424_1.html.

Bagchi, Sanjit. 2006. "Telemedicine in Rural India." *PLoS Medicine* 3 (3): 0297–99. https://
doi.org/10.1371/journal.pmed.0030082.

Balarajan, Yarlini, Selvaraj Selvaraj, and S. V. Subramanian. 2011. "Health Care and
Equity in India." *Lancet* 377 (9764): 505–15. https://doi.org/10.1016/S0140-6736
(10)61894-6.

Bamford, David R., and Paul L. Forrester. 2003. "Managing Planned and Emergent
Change within an Operations Management Environment." *International Journal
of Operations & Production Management* 23 (5): 546–64. https://doi.org/10.1108
/01443570310471857.

Banerjee, Dwaipayan. 2017. "Markets and Molecules: A Pharmaceutical Primer from
the South." *Medical Anthropology* 36 (4): 363–80. https://doi.org/10.1080/01459
740.2016.1209499.

Banik, Arindam, and Tirthankar Nag. 2016. "Bharti Airtel and Zain: A Journey into
New Territories." *Global Business Review* 17 (6): 1510–15. https://doi.org/10.1177
/0972150916660648.

Banik, Dan, and Emma Mawdsley. 2023. "South-South Cooperation and Global Development in a Multipolar World: China and India in Africa." *Journal of International
Development* 35: 539–48. https://doi.org/10.1002/jid.3789.

Banik, Dan, Meera Venkatachalam, and Renu Modi. 2023. *Catalysing Progress through Capacity-Building Initiatives: Learnings from India's Pan-African e-Network Project in Ghana and Malawi.* ORF Occasional Research Paper No. 420, Observer Research Foundation. https://www.orfonline.org/wp-content/uploads/2023/11/ORF _OP-420_Indias-capacity-building-initiatives-in-Africa.pdf.

Barad, Karen. 2003. "Posthumanist Performativity: Toward an Understanding of How Matter Comes to Matter." *Signs: Journal of Women in Culture* 28 (3): 801–31. https://doi.org/10.1086/345321.

Barad, Karen. 2007. *Meeting the Universe Halfway: Quantum Physics and the Entanglement of Matter and Meaning.* Durham, NC: Duke University Press.

Barker, Joshua. 2005. "Engineers and Political Dreams: Indonesia in the Satellite Age." *Current Anthropology* 46 (5): 703–27. https://doi.org/10.1086/432652.

Bärnreuther, Sandra. 2021. *Substantial Relations: Making Global Reproductive Medicine in Postcolonial India.* Ithaca, NY: Cornell University Press.

Baru, Rama V. 2018. "Medical-Industrial Complex: Trends in Corporatization of Health Services." In *Equity and Access: Health Care Studies in India*, edited by Purendra Prasad and Amar Jesani, 75–89. New Delhi, India: Oxford University Press.

Bashshur, R. L., and G. W. Shannon. 2009. *The History of Telemedicine: Evolution, Context, and Transformation.* New Rochelle, NY: Mary Ann Liebert.

Bazin, Bénédicte. 2019. "Étude d'une nouvelle forme de relation partenariale Sud-Sud influencée par les nouvelles technologies." Master in population and development sciences, Faculté des Sciences Sociales, Université de Liège. http://hdl.han dle.net/2268.2/8396.

Bear, Laura, Ritu Birla, and Stine Puri. 2015. "Speculation: Futures and Capitalism in India." *Comparative Studies of South Asia, Africa and the Middle East* 35 (3): 387–91. https://doi.org/10.1215/1089201X-3426241.

Bennett, Jane. 2010. *Vibrant Matter: A Political Ecology of Things.* Durham, NC: Duke University Press.

Beri, Ruchita. 2003. "India's Africa Policy in the Post-Cold War Era: An Assesment." *Strategic Analysis* 27 (2): 216–32. https://doi.org/10.1080/09700160308450084.

Berlant, Lauren. 2011. *Cruel Optimism.* Durham, NC: Duke University Press.

Berlant, Lauren. 2016. "The Commons: Infrastructures for Troubling Times." *Environment and Planning D: Society and Space* 34 (3): 393–419. https://doi.org/10.1177 /0263775816645989.

Bhagavan, Manu. 2017. "Reflections on Indian Internationalism and a Postnational Global Order: A Response to Partha Chatterjee." *Comparative Studies of South Asia, Africa and the Middle East* 37 (2): 220–25. https://doi.org/10.1215/1089201x-4132845.

Bhaskaranarayana, A., L. S. Satyamurthy, and Murthy Remilla. 2009. "Indian Space Research Organization and Telemedicine in India." *Telemedicine and e-Health* 15 (6): 586–91. https://doi.org/10.1089/tmj.2009.0060.

Bhatia, Rajiv. 2016. "The *Arthashastra* in Modi's India." In *Where Geopolitics Meets Business*, edited by Gateway House, 3–7. Mumbai, India: Gateway House: India Council on Global Relations.

Bhattacharya, Sanjukta Banerji. 2010. "Engaging Africa: India's interests in the African Continent, Past and Present." In *The Rise of China & India in Africa*, edited by Fantu Cheru and Cyril Obi, 63–76. London: Zed.

Bhushan, K., and G. Katyal. 2004. *Visionary to Certainty.* New Delhi, India: A. P. H.

Biao, Xiang. 2007. *Global "Body Shopping": An Indian Labor System in the Information Technology Industry.* Princeton, NJ: Princeton University Press.

Biehl, João, and Peter Locke, eds. 2017. *Unfinished: The Anthropology of Becoming.* Durham, NC: Duke University Press.

Bijoy, C. R. 2010. "India: Transiting to a Global Donor." In *South-South Cooperation: A Challenge to the Aid System?*, edited by The Reality of Aid, 65–76. Quezon City, Philippines: IBON.

Biruk, Crystal. 2018. *Cooking Data: Culture and Politics in an African Research World*. Durham, NC: Duke University Press.

Bochaton, Audrey, and Bertrand Lefebvre. 2008. "The Rebirth of the Hospital: Heterotopia and Medical Tourism in Asia." In *Asia on Tour*, edited by Tim Winter, Peggy Teo, and T. C. Chang, 113–24. London: Routledge.

Bowker, Geoffrey. 1995. "Second Nature Once Removed: Time, Space and Representations." *Time & Society* 4 (1): 47–66. https://doi.org/10.1177/0961463X950040 01003.

Bowker, Geoffrey, and Susan Leigh Star. 1999. *Sorting Things Out: Classification and Its Consequences*. Cambridge, MA: MIT Press.

Boyer, Dominic. 2010. "From Algos to Autonomos: Nostalgic Eastern Europe as Postimperial Mania." In *Post-communist Nostalgia*, edited by Maria Todorova and Zsuzsa Gille, 18–27. New York: Berghahn.

Brada, Betsey. 2011. "'Not Here': Making the Spaces and Subjects of 'Global Health' in Botswana." *Culture, Medicine, and Psychiatry* 35 (2): 285–312. https://doi.org/10 .1007/s11013-011-9209-z.

Braun, Bruce, and Sarah J. Whatmore, eds. 2010. *Political Matter: Technoscience, Democracy, and Public Life*. Minneapolis: Minnesota University Press.

Brewster, Liz, Gail Mountain, Bridgette Wessels, Ciara Kelly, and Mark Hawley. 2014. "Factors Affecting Front Line Staff Acceptance of Telehealth Technologies: A Mixed-Method Systematic Review." *Journal of Advanced Nursing* 70 (1): 21–33. https://doi.org/10.1111/jan.12196.

Brousse, V., P. Imbert, P. Mbaye, F. Kieffer, M. Thiam, A. S. Ka, P. Gerardin, and D. Sidi. 2003. "Evaluation au Sénégal du devenir des enfants transférés pour chirurgie cardiaque." *Médecine tropicale* 63 (4–5): 506–12.

Bryant, Levi, Nick Srnicek, and Graham Harman, eds. 2011. *The Speculative Turn: Continental Materialism and Realism*. Melbourne, Australia: re.press.

BT Bureau. 2015. "TCIL: Connecting the World via e-Network." *Bureaucracy Today*, May 6.

Burnes, Bernard. 2004. *Managing Change: A Strategic Approach to Organisational Dynamics*, 7th ed. Harlow, UK: Pearson Education.

Business Line. 2001. "Apollo Hospitals to Focus on Telemedicine." *Business Line (The Hindu)*, June 20.

BW Online Bureau. 2012. "The Last Frontier." *BW Businessworld*. October 15. https:// web.archive.org/web/20190203134143/http://www.businessworld.in/article /The-Last-Frontier/08-11-2014-67824/.

By, Rune Todnem. 2005. "Organisational Change Management: A Critical Review." *Journal of Change Management* 5 (4): 369–80. https://doi.org/10.1080/14697010500 359250.

Calkins, Sandra. 2021. "Toxic Remains: Infrastructural Failure in a Ugandan Molecular Biology Lab." *Social Studies of Science* 51 (5): 707–28. https://doi.org/10.1177 /03063127211011531.

Callén, Blanca, and Tomás Sánchez Criado. 2016. "Vulnerability Tests: Matters of 'Care for Matter' in E-waste Practices." *TECNOSCIENZA: Italian Journal of Science* 6 (2): 17–40. https://doi.org/10.6092/issn.2038-3460/17252.

Carr, E. Summerson, and Michael Lempert. 2016. "Introduction: Pragmatics of Scale." In *Scale: Discourse and Dimensions of Social Life*, edited by E. Summerson Carr and Michael Lempert, 1–21. Oakland: University of California Press.

Cartwright, Lisa. 2000. "Reach Out and Heal Someone: Telemedicine and the Glo-balization of Health Care." *Health* 4 (3): 347–77. https://doi.org/10.1177/1363 45930000400306.

CBHI. 2008. *Health Infrastructure, National Health Profile (NHP) of India–2008*. New Delhi: Central Bureau of Health Intelligence, Government of India.

Chakrabarty, Dipesh. 2000. *Provincializing Europe: Postcolonial Thought and Historical Difference*. Princeton, NJ: Princeton University Press.

Chakrabarty, Dipesh. 2005. "Legacies of Bandung: Decolonisation and the Politics of Culture." *Economic and Political Weekly* 40 (46): 4812–18. https://www.jstor.org /stable/4417389.

Chakravartty, Paula. 2012. "Rebranding Development Communications in Emergent India." *Nordicum Review* (33): 65–76. https://doi.org/10.2478/nor-2013-0026.

Chamayou, Grégoire. 2015. *A Theory of the Drone*. New York: New Press.

Chand, Manish. 2011. "Skill Development: The ITEC Way." In *Two Billion Dreams . . . Celebrating India-Africa Friendship*, edited by Manish Chand, 111–20. Delhi, India: IANS.

Chatterjee, Partha. 2016. "Nationalism, Internationalism, and Cosmopolitanism: Some Observations from Modern Indian History." *Comparative Studies of South Asia, Africa and the Middle East* 36 (2): 320–34. https://doi.org/10.1215/1089201X-36 03392.

Chatterjee, Partha. 2017. "Empires, Nations, Peoples: The Imperial Prerogative and Colonial Exceptions." *Thesis Eleven* 139 (1): 84–96. https://doi.org/10.1177/07 25513617700040.

Chattu, V. K., B. Singh, F. Kajal, C. Chatla, S. K. Chattu, S. Pattanshetty, and K. S. Reddy. 2023. "The Rise of India's Global Health Diplomacy Amid COVID-19 Pandemic." *Health Promotion Perspectives* 13 (4): 290–98. https://doi.org/10.34172/hpp .2023.34.

Chen, Kuan-Hsing. 2010. *Asia as Method: Toward Deimperialization*. Durham, NC: Duke University Press.

Chhabra, Hari Sharan. 1989. *Nehru and Resurgent Africa*. New Delhi, India: Africa Publications.

Chib, Arul. 2013. "The Promise and Peril of mHealth in Developing Countries." *Mobile Media & Communication* 1 (1): 69–75. https://doi.org/10.1177/2050157912459502.

Chinai, Rupa, and Rahul Goswami. 2007. "Medical Visas Mark Growth of Indian Medi-cal Tourism." *Bulletin of the World Health Organization* 85 (3): 164–65. https:// doi.org/10.2471/BLT.07.010307.

Chopra, Rohit. 2008. *Technology and Nationalism in India: Cultural Negociations from Colonialism to Cyberspace*. Amherst, NY: Cambia.

Chun, Wendy Hui Kyong. 2015. "Networks NOW: Belated Too Early." In *Postdigital Aesthetics: Art, Computation and Design*, edited by David M. Berry and Michael Dieter, 289–315. New York: Palgrave Macmillan.

Chun, Wendy Hui Kyong, and Jorge Cotte. 2020. "Reimagining Networks: An Interview with Wendy Hui Kyong Chun." *New Inquiry*, May 12. https://thenewinquiry.com /reimagining-networks.

Clarke, Sir Arthur. 2004. "Foreword: Communications for Goodness' Sake." In *Promot-ing ICT for Human Development in Asia 2004: Realising the Millennium Develop-ment Goals*, edited by United Nations Development Programme. New Delhi, India: Elsevier.

Connell, John. 2006. "Medical Tourism: Sea, Sun, Sand and . . . Surgery." *Tourism Man-agement* 27 (6): 1093–1100. https://doi.org/10.1016/j.tourman.2005.11.005.

Connolly, William E. 2011. *A World of Becoming*. Durham, NC: Duke University Press.

Connor, Steven. 2002. "Topologies: Michel Serres and the Shapes of Thought." Accessed May 27, 2024. http://stevenconnor.com/topologies.html.

Coole, Diana, and Samantha Frost, eds. 2010. *New Materialisms: Ontology, Agency, and Politics*. Durham, NC: Duke University Press.

Cross, Jamie. 2014. *Dream Zones: Anticipating Capitalism and Development in India*. London: Pluto.

Das, Gurcharan. 2002. *India Unbound*. New York: Anchor.

Das, S. K. 2007. *Touching Lives: The Little Known Triumphs of the Indian Space Programme*. New Delhi, India: Penguin.

De Bruyn, Tom. 2018. "Equal Relations and Appropriate Expertise in India's South-South Co-Operation? Discourse and Practice of the Pan-African e-Network." *Insight on Africa* 10 (1): 1–20. https://doi.org/10.1177/0975087817735384.

de Jacquelot, Patrick. 2011. "L'Inde, l'autre grande soeur de l'Afrique." *Les Echos*, 23 mai 2011, 10. https://www.lesechos.fr/2011/05/linde-lautre-grande-soeur-de-laf rique-1089985.

Deleuze, Gilles. 1988. *Foucault*. Translated by Sean Hand. Minneapolis: University of Minnesota Press.

Denis, David J. 2019. "Why Do Maintenance and Repair Matter?" In *The Routledge Companion to Actor-Network Theory*, edited by Anders Blok, Ignacio Farías, and Celia Roberts, 283–93. New York: Routledge.

Denis, Jérôme, and David Pontille. 2015. "Material Ordering and the Care of Things." *Science, Technology, Human Values* 40 (3): 338–67. https://doi.org/10.1177/01622 43914553129.

Devarakonda, Srichand. 2016. "Hub and Spoke Model: Making Rural Healthcare in India Affordable, Available and Accessible." *Rural and Remote Health* 16 (1): 1–8. https://doi.org/10.22605/RRH3476.

Diagne, Souleymane Bachir. 2013. "On the Postcolonial and the Universal?" *Rue Descartes* 78 (2): 7–18. https://doi.org/10.3917/rdes.078.0007.

Diagne, Souleymane Bachir. 2017. "Pour un universel vraiment universel." In *Écrire l'Afrique-monde*, edited by Achille Mbembe and Felwine Sarr, 73–78. Dakar, Senegal: Philippe Rey.

Dihel, Nora, and Arti Grover Goswami. 2016. *The Unexplored Potential of Trade in Services in Africa*. Washington, DC: World Bank. https://documents1.worldbank.org /curated/en/477321469182630728/pdf/107185-WP-TradeinServiceWeb-PUBLIC .pdf.

Dilger, Hansjörg, Abdoulaye Kane, and Stacey A. Langwick. 2012. *Medicine, Mobility, and Power in Global Africa: Transnational Health and Healing*. Bloomington: Indiana University Press.

Dilger, Hansjörg, and Dominik Mattes. 2018. "Im/Mobilities and Dis/Connectivities in Medical Globalisation: How Global Is Global Health?" *Global Public Health* 13 (3): 265–75. https://doi.org/10.1080/17441692.2017.1414285.

Diouf, Mamadou. 1999. "Introduction. Entre l'Afrique et l'Inde: sur les questions coloniales et nationales. Ecritures de l'histoire et recherches historiques." In *L'historiographe indienne en débat: colonialisme, nationalisme et sociétés postcoloniales*, edited by Mamadou Diouf, 5–35. Paris: Éditions Karthala et Sephis.

Dubey, Ajay Kumar. 1991. *Indo-African Relations in the Post-Nehru Era*. Delhi, India: Kalinga.

Duclos, Vincent. 2012. "Building Capacities: The Resurgence of Indo-African Techno-economic Cooperation." *India Review* 11 (4): 209–25. https://doi.org/10.1080/1 4736489.2012.731906.

Duclos, Vincent. 2015. "Global eHealth: Designing Spaces of Care in the Era of Global Connectivity." *Medicine Anthropology Theory* 2 (1): 154–64. https://doi.org/10 .17157/mat.2.1.166.

Duclos, Vincent. 2017. "Demanding Mobile Health." *Limn* 9: 17–21. https://limn.it/arti cles/demanding-mobile-health.

Duclos, Vincent. 2019a. "Algorithmic Futures: The Life and Death of Google Flu Trends." *Medicine Anthropology Theory* 6 (3): 54–76. https://doi.org/10.17157/mat.6.3.660.

Duclos, Vincent. 2019b. "Falling into Things: Peter Sloterdijk, Ontological Anthropology in the Monstrous." *New Formations* 95: 37–53. https://doi.org/10.3898/nEW F:95.03.2018.

Duclos, Vincent, and Tomás Sánchez Criado. 2020. "Care in Trouble: Ecologies of Support from Below & Beyond." *Medical Anthropology Quarterly* 34 (2): 153–73. https://doi .org/10.1111/maq.12540.

Duclos, Vincent, Tomás Sánchez Criado, and Vinh-Kim Nguyen. 2017. "Speed: An Introduction." *Cultural Anthropology* 32 (1): 1–11. https://doi.org/10.14506/ca 32.1.01.

Dyer, Owen. 2023. "Covid-19: Drug Companies Charged South Africa High Prices for Vaccines, Contracts Reveal." *BMJ* 382: p2112. https://doi.org/10.1136/bmj.p2112. https://www.bmj.com/content/bmj/382/bmj.p2112.full.pdf.

Easton, Alice. 2010. "NDM-1: Reactions from India." *One Health Trust* (blog). Last modified August 19, 2010. https://onehealthtrust.org/news-media/blog/ndm-1 -reactions-from-india.

Einhorn, Bruce. 2002. "India and IT: 'Like France and Wine.'" *BusinessWeek*, January 28. https://www.bloomberg.com/news/articles/2002-01-27/india-and-it-like-fra nce-and-wine?leadSource=uverify%20wall.

Elbert, Bruce R. 2004. *The Satellite Communication Applications Handbook.* Norwood, MA: Artech House.

Elrod, James K., and John L. Fortenberry. 2017. "The Hub-and-Spoke Organization Design: An Avenue for Serving Patients Well." *BMC Health Services Research* 17 (1): 25–33. https://doi.org/10.1186/s12913-017-2341-x.

Erikson, Susan. 2019. "Global Health Futures? Reckoning with a Pandemic Bond." *Medicine Anthropology Theory* 6 (3): 77–108. https://doi.org/10.17157/mat.6.3.664.

Express News Service. 2010. "Kalam Sees Human Habitats on Moon, Mars by 2050." *Indian Express*, June 2. http://www.indianexpress.com/news/kalam-sees-human -habitats-on-moon-mars-by-2050/628073.

Fall, Ndèye Khaïba. 2009. "TIC et développement au Sénégal: Enjeux et perspectives du marketing territorial de Dakar pour les téléservices." Master's thesis, Département de géographie, Université Cheikh Anta Diop. http://196.1.97.20/viewer.php? c=mmoires&d=meml%5f5928.

Farman, Abou, and Richard Rottenburg. 2019. "Measures of Future Health, from the Nonhuman to the Planetary." *Medicine Anthropology Theory* 6 (3): 1–28. https:// doi.org/10.17157/mat.6.3.659.

Farquhar, Judith. 2016. "The Fold (Magic Words: A Numbered List)." *Somatosphere.* Last modified March 21, 2016. http://somatosphere.net/2016/magic-words-a -numbered-list.html.

Ferguson, Earl W., Charles R. Doarn, and John C. Scott. 1995. "Survey of Global Telemedicine." *Journal of Medical Systems* 19 (1): 35–46. https://doi.org/10.1007/BF02257189.

Ferguson, James. 2006. *Global Shadows: Africa in the Neoliberal World Order.* Durham, NC: Duke University Press.

Final Communiqué. 2009. "Final Communiqué of the Asian-African Conference." *Interventions* 11 (1): 94–102. https://doi.org/10.1080/13698010902752830.

Fortun, Mike. 2008. *Promising Genomics: Iceland and deCODE Genetics in a World of Speculation.* Berkeley: University of California Press.

Foucault, Michel. 1969. *L'archéologie du savoir.* Paris: Gallimard.

Foucault, Michel. 1973. *The Birth of the Clinic: An Archaeology of Medical Perception.* Translated by A. M. Sheridan. London: Routledge.

Foucault, Michel. [2001] 1961. *Madness and Civilization: A History of Insanity in the Age of Reason.* Translated by Richard Howard. London: Routledge.

Fuller, Chris J., and Haripriya Narasimhan. 2007. "Information Technology Professionals and the New-Rich Middle Class in Chennai (Madras)." *Modern Asian Studies* 41 (1): 121–50. https://doi.org/10.1017/S0026749X05002325.

Fullsack, Jean-Louis. 2012. "La gouvernance discutable de l'UIT: Le projet Africa ONE comme exemple." *tic & société* 5 (2–3): 94–119. https://doi.org/10.4000/ticetso ciete.1089.

Gad, Christopher, Casper Bruun Jensen, and Brit Ross Winthereik. 2015. "Practical Ontology: Worlds in STS and Anthropology." *NatureCulture* 3: 67–86. https://doi .org/10.18910/75520.

Galloway, Alexander R., and Eugene Thacker. 2007. *The Exploit. A Theory of Networks.* Minneapolis: University of Minnesota Press.

Ganapathy, Krishnan, and Aditi Ravindra. 2009. "Telemedicine in India: The Apollo Story." *Telemedecine and e-Health* 15 (6): 576–85. https://doi.org/10.1089/tmj .2009.0066.

Geissbuhler, A., O. Ly, C. Lovis, and J. F. L'Haire. 2003. "Telemedicine in Western Africa: Lessons Learned from a Pilot Project in Mali, Perspectives and Recommendations." *AMIA Annual Symposium Proceedings* (2003): 249–53.

Geissler, P. Wenzel. 2014. "The Archipelago of Public Health: Comments on the Landscape of Medical Research in Twenty-First-Century Africa." In *Making and Unmaking Public Health in Africa: Ethnographic and Historical Perspectives*, edited by Ruth J. Prince and Rebecca Marsland, 231–56. Athens: Ohio University Press.

Geissler, P. Wenzel. 2015. *Para-States and Medical Science: Making African Global Health.* Durham, NC: Duke University Press.

Geissler, P. Wenzel, Ann Kelly, Babatunde Imoukhuede, and Robert Pool. 2008. "'He Is Now Like a Brother, I Can Even Give Him Some Blood'—Relational Ethics and Material Exchanges in a Malaria Vaccine 'Trial Community' in the Gambia." *Social Science & Medicine* 67 (5): 696–707. https://doi.org/10.1016/j.socscimed .2008.02.004.

Geissler, P. Wenzel, and Noémi Tousignant. 2020. "Beyond Realism: Africa's Medical Dreams. Introduction." *Africa* 90 (1): 1–17. https://doi.org/10.1017/S000197201 9000913.

Glissant, Édouard. 1997. *Poetics of Relation.* Ann Arbor: University of Michigan Press.

Godbout, Jacques T., and Alain C. Caille. 1998. *World of the Gift.* Montreal, Canada: McGill-Queen's Press-MQUP.

Godelier, Maurice. 1999. *The Enigma of the Gift.* Chicago: University of Chicago Press.

Goldberg, Allyson M. 2013. "Medical Tourism? A Case Study of African Patients in India." Master's thesis, University of California, Berkeley. https://escholarship.org /uc/item/89t9j2b8.

Government of India. 1964. *Ministry of External Affairs Annual Report.* Ministry of External Affairs. https://mealib.nic.in/?pdf2491?000.

Govindarajan, Vijay, and Ravi Ramamurti. 2013. "Delivering World-Class Health Care, Affordably." *Harvard Business Review* 91 (11): 117–22. https://hbr.org/2013/11 /delivering-world-class-health-care-affordably.

Graeber, David. 2001. *Toward an Anthropological Theory of Value: The False Coin of Our Own Dreams*. New York: Springer.

Graham, L. E., M. Zimmerman, D. J. Vassallo, V. Patterson, P. Swinfen, R. Swinfen, and R. Wootton. 2003. "Telemedicine—The Way Ahead for Medicine in the Developing World." *Tropical Doctor* 33 (1): 36–38. https://doi.org/10.1177/004947550 303300118.

Graham, Stephen, and Nigel Thrift. 2007. "Out of Order. Understanding Repair and Maintenance." *Theory, Culture & Society* 24 (3): 1–25. https://doi.org/10.1177/02 63276407075954.

Graziplene, Leonard R. 2009. *Creating Telemedicine-Based Medical Networks for Rural and Frontier Areas*. IBM Center for the Business of Government. https://www.businessofgovernment.org/sites/default/files/Creating%20telemedicine-based%20medicalpdf.pdf.

Greene, Jeremy A. 2022. *The Doctor Who Wasn't There: Technology, History, and the Limits of Telehealth*. Chicago: University of Chicago Press.

Greene, Jeremy A., Victor Braitberg, and Gabriella Maya Bernadett. 2020. "Innovation on the Reservation: Information Technology and Health Systems Research among the Papago Tribe of Arizona, 1965–1980." *Isis* 111 (3): 443–70. https://doi.org/10.1086/710802.

Greenspan, Anna. 2004. *India and the IT Revolution. Networks of Global Culture*. New York: Palgrave Macmillan.

Gregory, Chris A. 2015. *Gifts and Commodities*. Chicago: HAU.

Groves, Trish. 1996. "SatelLife: Getting Relevant Information to the Developing World." *British Medical Journal* 313 (7072): 1606–09. https://doi.org/10.1136/bmj.313.70 72.1606.

Guha, Ramachandra. 2012. "Indians Great, Greater, Greatest?" *The Hindu*. Last modified July 21, 2012. https://www.thehindu.com/opinion/op-ed/indians-great-greater -greatest/article3662823.ece.

Hall, Ian. 2017. "Modi's Vision for India as a Normative Power." *East Asia Forum*. Last modified February 8, 2017. https://www.eastasiaforum.org/2017/02/08/modis -vision-for-india-as-a-normative-power.

Haraway, Donna J. 2016. *Staying with the Trouble: Making Kin in the Chthulucene*. Durham, NC: Duke University Press.

Harman, Graham. 2018. *Object-Oriented Ontology: A New Theory of Everything*. London: Penguin UK.

Harvey, Brian. 2000. *The Japanese and Indian Space Programmes*. Chichester, UK: Praxis.

Harvey, Penelope, Christian Krohn-Hansen, and Knut G. Nustad. 2019. "Introduction." In *Anthropos and the Material*, edited by Penelope Harvey, Christian Krohn-Hansen, and Knut G. Nustad, 1–30. Durham, NC: Duke University Press.

Harvey, Penny, Casper Bruun Jensen, and Atsuro Morita. 2016. "Introduction: Infrastructural Complications." In *Infrastructures and Social Complexity*, 19–40. New York: Routledge.

Henke, Christopher R. 2000. "The Mechanics of Workplace Order: Toward a Sociology of Repair." *Berkeley Journal of Sociology* 44: 55–81. http://www.jstor.org/stable /41035546.

Hersh, Seymour M. 1983. *The Price of Power: Kissinger in the Nixon White House*. New York: Summit Books.

Hirschkind, Charles, Maria José A. de Abreu, and Carlo Caduff. 2017. "New Media, New Publics? An Introduction to Supplement 15." *Current Anthropology* 58 (S15): S3–S12. https://doi.org/10.1086/688903.

Hofmeyr, Isabel. 2018. "Against the Global South." In *The Global South and Literature*, edited by Russell West-Pavlov, 307–14. Cambridge, UK: Cambridge University Press.

Holst, Christine, Felix Sukums, Danica Radovanovic, Bernard Ngowi, Josef Noll, and Andrea Sylvia Winkler. 2020. "Sub-Saharan Africa—The New Breeding Ground for Global Digital Health." *Lancet Digital Health* 2 (4): e160–e162. https://doi .org/10.1016/S2589-7500(20)30027-3.

Hope, Jenny. 2010. "Alarm over 'Unbeatable' Enzyme That Could Make All Bacterial Diseases Resistant to Antibiotics." *Daily Mail*, August 12. https://www.dailymail .co.uk/health/article-1302035/Unbeatable-NDM-1-enzyme-make-bacterial-dis eases-superbugs.html.

Hu, Tung-Hui. 2015. *A Prehistory of the Cloud*. Cambridge, MA: MIT Press.

Huang, Fei, Sean Blaschke, and Henry Lucas. 2017. "Beyond Pilotitis: Taking Digital Health Interventions to the National Level in China and Uganda." *Globalization and Health* 13 (1): 49. https://doi.org/10.1186/s12992-017-0275-z.

IMTJ. 2016. "Africa Spends $1 Billion a Year on Outbound Medical Tourism." *IMTJ*, August 3. https://www.laingbuissonnews.com/imtj/news-imtj/africa-spends-1-bil lion-a-year-on-outbound-medical-tourism.

India Africa Connect. 2012. "Health in India: An Overview." Accessed October 18, 2024. https://indiaafricaconnect.in/index.php?param=categorydetails/health-edu cation/106.

Ingold, Tim. 2006. "Rethinking the Animate, Re-Animating Thought." *Ethnos* 71 (1): 9–20. https://doi.org/10.1080/00141840600603111.

Ingold, Tim. 2007. *Lines. A Brief History*. London: Routledge.

Ingold, Tim. 2011. *Being Alive: Essays on Movement, Knowledge and Description*. London: Routledge.

International Institute for Population Sciences (IIPS) and ORC Macro. 2000. *National Family Health Survey (NFHS-2), 1998–99: India*. Mumbai, India: IIPS.

Irani, Lilly. 2019. *Chasing Innovation: Making Entrepreneurial Citizens in Modern India*. Princeton, NJ: Princeton University Press.

Irani, Lilly, and Kavita Philip. 2018. "Negotiating Engines of Difference." *Catalyst: Feminism, Theory, Technoscience* 4 (2): 1–11. https://doi.org/10.28968/cftt.v4i2.29841.

Jackson, Steven J., Alex Pompe, and Gabriel Krieshok. 2012. "Repair Worlds: Maintenance, Repair, and ICT For Development in Rural Namibia." Proceedings of the ACM 2012 conference on Computer Supported Cooperative Work, Seattle. https://doi.org/10.1145/2145204.2145224.

Jackson, Zakiyyah Iman. 2018. "'Theorizing in a Void': Sublimity, Matter, and Physics in Black Feminist Poetics." *South Atlantic Quarterly* 117 (3): 617–48.

Jain, Devaki. 2016. "Looking Back at the South Commission." *Economic & Political Weekly* 51 (9): 62–66.

Jaishankar, Subrahmanyam. 2020. *The India Way: Strategies for an Uncertain World*. New Delhi, India: HarpersCollins.

Jeffrey, Craig. 2010. *Timepass: Youth, Class, and the Politics of Waiting in India*. Stanford, CA: Stanford University Press.

Jensen, Casper Bruun. 2006. "Technologic: Conceptualising Health Care Transformation with the Electronic Patient Record." *Systems, Signs & Actions* 2 (1): 41–59.

Jensen, Casper Bruun. 2010. *Ontologies for Developing Things*. Rotterdam, The Netherlands: Sense.

Johny, Stanly. 2013. "Heading Due South." *Business Standard*, June 17. https://www .business-standard.com/article/beyond-business/heading-due-south-113061 600611_1.html.

Joseph, Justin Jada. 2012. "South Sudan Soon to Launch Tele-Education and Medicine." *AllAfrica*, October 4. https://allafrica.com/stories/201210040258.html.

Juma, Calestous, and Elisabeth Moyer. 2008. "Broadband Internet for Africa." *Science* 320 (5881): 1261. https://doi.org/10.1126/science.1161105.

Kalam, Abdul. 2003. *Ignited Minds: Unleashing the Power Within India*. New Delhi, India: Penguin Global.

Kalam, Abdul. 2007. *Indomitable Spirit*. New Delhi, India: Rajpal.

Kalam, Abdul. 2011. *Building a New India*. New Delhi, India: Penguin.

Kalam, Abdul, and A. Sivathanu Pillai. 2004. *Envisioning an Empowered Nation: Technology for Societal Transformation*. New Delhi, India: Tata McGraw-Hill.

Kamat, Sangeeta. 2004. "Postcolonial Aporias, or What Does Fundamentalism Have to Do with Globalization? The Contradictory Consequences of Education Reform in India." *Comparative Education* 40 (2): 267–87. https://doi.org/10.1080/03050 06042000231383.

Kane, Oumar. 2010. *L'organisation des télécommunications au Sénégal: Entre gouvernance et régulation*. Paris: Éditions Karthala.

Kapoor, Ilan. 2008. *The Postcolonial Politics of Development*, 1st ed. London: Routledge.

Kaspar, Heidi, Margaret Walton-Roberts, and Audrey Bochaton. 2019. "Therapeutic Mobilities." *Mobilities* 14 (1): 1–19. https://doi.org/10.1080/17450101.2019.1565305.

Katti, Vijaya, Tatjana Chahoud, and Atul Kaushik. 2009. "India's Development Cooperation—Opportunities and Challenges for International Development Cooperation." German Development Institute. http://www.die-gdi.de/CMS-Homepage /openwebcms3.nsf/%28ynDK_contentByKey%29/ANES-7QAGRV?Open.

Kaur, Ravinder. 2020. *Brand New Nation: Capitalist Dreams and Nationalist Designs in Twenty-First-Century India*. Stanford, CA: Stanford University Press.

Kaur, Ravinder, and Thomas Blom Hansen. 2016. "Aesthetics of Arrival: Spectacle, Capital, Novelty in Post-Reform India." *Identities* 23 (3): 265–75. https://doi.org/10.1 080/1070289X.2015.1034135.

Kelly, Ann H., and Linsey McGoey. 2018. "Facts, Power and Global Evidence: A New Empire of Truth." *Economy and Society* 47 (1): 1–26. https://doi.org/10.1080/030 85147.2018.1457261.

Kenworthy, Nora J. 2014. "Global Health: The Debts of Gratitude." *Women's Studies Quarterly* 42 (1/2): 69–85.

Kithuure, Julius. 2014. "Kenya's Plan to Build High-End Medical Centres Draws Mixed Reviews." *allAfrica*, December 4. https://allafrica.com/stories/201412050187.html.

Kragelund, Peter. 2010. *The Potential Role of Non-Traditional Donors' Aid in Africa*. Issue Paper No. 11, International Centre for Trade and Sustainable Development (Geneva, Switzerland). https://www.files.ethz.ch/isn/113430/2010_03_the-poten tial-role-of-non-traditional-donorse28099-aid-in-africa.pdf.

Krishnan, Vidya. 2024. "India's 'Whitey on the Moon' Moment." *Al Jazeera*, February 22. https://www.aljazeera.com/opinions/2024/2/22/indias-whitey-on-the-moon -moment.

Kumar, Girish. 2009. "Introduction: Health Sector Reforms in India: Issues, Experiences and Trends." In *Health Sector Reforms in India*, edited by Girish Kumar, 13–44. New Delhi, India: CSH-Manohar.

Kumar, Shailender. 2015. *Private Sector in Health Care Delivery Market in India: Structure, Growth and Implications*. Working Paper 185, Institute for Studies in Industrial Development (New Delhi). https://ideas.repec.org/p/sid/wpaper/185.html.

Kumarasamy, Karthikeyan K., Mark A. Toleman, Timothy R. Walsh, Jay Bagaria, Fafhana Butt, Ravikumar Balakrishnan, Uma Chaudhary, Michel Doumith, Christian G. Giske, and Seema Irfan. 2010. "Emergence of a New Antibiotic Resistance Mechanism in India, Pakistan, and the UK: A Molecular, Biological, and Epidemiological Study." *Lancet Infectious Diseases* 10 (9): 597–602. https://doi.org/10.1016/S1473-3099(10)70143-2.

Labrique, Alain B., Christina Wadhwani, Koku Awoonor Williams, Peter Lamptey, Cees Hesp, Rowena Luk, and Ann Aerts. 2018. "Best Practices in Scaling Digital Health in Low and Middle Income Countries." *Globalization and Health* 14 (1): 103. https://doi.org/10.1186/s12992-018-0424-z.

Larkin, Brian. 2013. "The Politics and Poetics of Infrastructure." *Annual Review of Anthropology* 42 (1): 327–43. https://doi.org/10.1146/annurev-anthro-092412-155522.

Latour, Bruno. 1993. *We Have Never Been Modern*. Cambridge, MA: Harvard University Press.

Latour, Bruno. 1996. *Aramis, or the Love of Technology*. Cambridge, MA: Harvard University Press.

Latour, Bruno. 2004. "Why Has Critique Run Out of Steam? From Matters of Fact to Matters of Concern." *Critical Inquiry* 30 (2): 225–48.

Latour, Bruno. 2007a. "Can We Get Our Materialism Back, Please?" *Isis* 98 (1): 138–42. https://doi.org/10.1086/512837.

Latour, Bruno. 2007b. "How to Think Like a State." Lecture delivered on November 22, 2007 at the occasion of the anniversary of the WRR in presence of Queen Beatrix of The Netherlands. http://www.bruno-latour.fr/sites/default/files/P-133-LA%20HAYE-QUEEN.pdf.

Latour, Bruno. 2008. "A Cautious Prometheus? A Few Steps Toward a Philosophy of Design (With Special Attention to Peter Sloterdijk)." In *Proceedings of the 2008 Annual International Conference of the Design History Society*, edited by Fiona Hackne, Jonathan Glynne, and Viv Minto, 2–10. Falmouth, MA: Universal.

Latour, Bruno, Graham Harman, and Peter Erdélyi. 2011. *The Prince and the Wolf: Latour and Harman at the LSE*. Hants, UK: Zero.

Law, John. 1999. "After ANT: Complexity, Naming and Topology." *Sociological Review* 47 (S1): 1–14. https://doi.org/10.1111/j.1467-954X.1999.tb03479.x.

Law, John, and Marianne Elisabeth Lien. 2013. "Slippery: Field Notes in Empirical Ontology." *Social Studies of Science* 43 (3): 363–78. https://doi.org/10.1177/0306312712456947.

Leblanc, Jacques G. 2009. "Creating a Global Climate for Pediatric Cardiac Care." *World Journal of Pediatrics* 5 (2): 89–92. https://doi.org/10.1007/s12519-009-0019-0.

Lee, Christopher J. 2010. "Introduction. Between a Moment and an Era: The Origins and Afterlives of Bandung." In *Making a World after Empire: The Bandung Moment and Its Political Afterlives*, edited by Christopher J. Lee, 1–42. Athens: Ohio University Press.

Lefebvre, Bertrand. 2010. "Hospital Chains in India. The Coming of Age?" Janvier 2010, IFRI. http://hal.archives-ouvertes.fr/docs/00/68/71/05/PDF/IFRI_asievisions23blefebvre.pdf.

Le Monde. 2007. "La fusée Ariane 5 a lancé le premier satellite panafricain." *Le Monde*, 22 décembre 2007. http://www.lemonde.fr/planete/article/2007/12/22/la-fusee-ariane-5-a-lance-le-premier-satellite-panafricain_992580_3244.html.

Livingston, Julie. 2012. *Improvising Medicine: An African Oncology Ward in an Emerging Cancer Epidemic*. Durham, NC: Duke University Press.

Lock, Margaret, and Vinh-Kim Nguyen. 2018. *An Anthropology of Biomedicine*, 2nd ed. Oxford, UK: John Wiley & Sons.

Lorway, Robert. 2017. "Making Global Health Knowledge: Documents, Standards, and Evidentiary Sovereignty in HIV Interventions in South India." *Critical Public Health* 27 (2): 177–92. https://doi.org/10.1080/09581596.2016.1262941.

Ly, Birama Apho, Ronald Labonté, Ivy Lynn Bourgeault, and Mbayang Ndiaye Niang. 2017. "The Individual and Contextual Determinants of the Use of Telemedicine: A Descriptive Study of the Perceptions of Senegal's Physicians and Telemedicine Projects Managers." *PLOS ONE* 12 (7): e0181070. https://doi.org/10.1371/journal .pone.0181070.

Mackenzie, Adrian. 2010. *Wirelessness: Radical Empiricism in Network Cultures*. Cambridge, MA: MIT Press.

MacReady, Norra. 2007. "Developing Countries Court Medical Tourists." *Lancet* 369 (9576): 1849–50. https://doi.org/10.1016/S0140-6736(07)60833-2.

Mahajan, Manjari. 2019. "The IHME in the Shifting Landscape of Global Health Metrics." *Global Policy* 10: 110–20. https://doi.org/10.1111/1758-5899.12605.

Mahal, Ajay, Bibek Debroy, and Laveesh Bandhari. 2010. *India Health Report 2010*. Indicus Analytics. New Delhi, India: Business Standard Limited.

Mair, Frances, Tracy Finch, Carl May, Julia Hiscock, Susan Beaton, Pauline Goldstein, and Siobhann McQuillan. 2007. "Perceptions of Risk as a Barrier to the Use of Telemedicine." *Journal of Telemedicine and Telecare* 13 (1_suppl): 38–39. https://doi.org /10.1258/135763307781645158.

Malecki, Edward J., and Hu Wei. 2009. "A Wired World: The Evolving Geography of Submarine Cables and the Shift to Asia." *Annals of the Association of American Geographers* 99 (2): 360–82. https://doi.org/10.1080/00045600802686216.

Martínez, Francisco, and Patrick Laviolette, eds. 2019. *Repair, Brokenness, Breakthrough: Ethnographic Responses*. New York: Berghahn.

Marx, Karl. [1906] 1867. *Capital: A Critique of Political Economy*. New York: Random House.

Massumi, Brian. 2002. *Parables for the Virtual: Movement, Affect, Sensation*. Durham, NC: Duke University Press.

Mauss, Marcel. [2002] 1925. *The Gift*. Translated by J. I. Guyer. London: Routledge.

Mavhunga, Clapperton Chakanetsa. 2017. "Introduction: What Do Science, Technology, and Innovation Mean from Africa?" In *What Do Science, Technology, and Innovation Mean from Africa?*, edited by Clapperton Chakanetsa Mavhunga, 1–27. Cambridge, MA: MIT Press.

Mawdsley, Emma. 2011. "The Rhetorics and Rituals of 'South-South' Development Cooperation: Notes on India and Africa." In *India in Africa: Changing Geographies of Power*, edited by Emma Mawdsley and Gerard McCann, 166–86. Oxford, UK: Pambazuka.

Mawdsley, Emma. 2012. "The Changing Geographies of Foreign Aid and Development Cooperation: Contributions from Gift Theory." *Transactions of the Institute of British Geographers* 37 (2): 256–72. https://doi.org/10.1111/j.1475-5661.2011.00467.x.

Mazzarella, William. 2010. "Beautiful Balloon: The Digital Divide and the Charisma of New Media in India." *American Ethnologist* 37 (4): 783–804. https://doi.org/10.11 11/j.1548-1425.2010.01285.x.

Mazzarella, William. 2012. "'Reality Must Improve': The Perversity of Expertise and the Belatedness of Indian Development Television." *Global Media and Communication* 8 (3): 215–41. https://doi.org/10.1177/1742766512459120.

Mazzarella, William. 2017. *The Mana of Mass Society*. Chicago: University of Chicago Press.

Mazzarella, William. 2019. "Brand(ish)ing the Name; or, Why Is Trump So Enjoyable?" In *Sovereignty, Inc.: Three Inquiries in Politics and Enjoyment*, edited by William Mazzarella, Eric L. Santner, and Aaron Schuster, 113–60. Chicago: University of Chicago Press.

Mazzarella, William. 2022. "Charisma in the Age of Trumpism." *e-flux Notes*, September 22. https://www.e-flux.com/notes/492472/charisma-in-the-age-of-trumpism.

Mbembe, Achille. 2012. "Theory from the Antipodes: Notes on Jean & John Coma-roffs' TFS. Theorizing the Contemporary, Fieldsights." *Cultural Anthropology*, February 25. https://culanth.org/fieldsights/theory-from-the-antipodes-notes-on-jean-john-comaroffs-tfs.

Mbembe, Achille. 2017. *Critique of Black Reason.* Durham, NC: Duke University Press.

Mbembe, Achille. 2018. "The Idea of a Borderless World." *Africa Is a Country* (blog). November 11. https://africasacountry.com/2018/11/the-idea-of-a-borderless-world.

Mbembe, Achille, and Bregtje van der Haak. 2015. "The Internet Is Afropolitan." This Is Africa (TIA). https://thisisafrica.me/politics-and-society/the-internet-is-afropolitan/.

McCann, Gerard. 2013. "From Diaspora to Third Worldism and the United Nations: India and the Politics of Decolonizing Africa." *Past & Present* 218 (suppl_8): 258–80. https://doi.org/10.1093/pastj/gts043.

McKay, Ramah. 2019. "Beyond the Pharmaceutical South: The Many Transnationalism of Medicine in Mozambique." Unpublished work.

McKenna, Maryn. 2010. "The 'Indian Superbug': Worse Than We Knew." *Wired*, September 14. https://www.wired.com/2010/09/the-indian-superbug-worse-than-we-knew/.

McLuhan, Marshall. 1966. "The Emperor's Old Clothes." In *The Man-Made Object*, edited by Gyorgy Kepes, 90–95. New York: Braziller.

McLuhan, Marshall. 2003. *Understanding Media: The Extensions of Man.* Berkeley, CA: Gingko.

Meier zu Biesen, Caroline. 2018. "From Coastal to Global: The Transnational Flow of Ayurveda and Its Relevance for Indo-African Linkages." *Global Public Health* 13 (3): 339–54. https://doi.org/10.1080/17441692.2017.1281328.

Menon, Dilip M. 2014. "Bandung Is Back: Afro-Asian Affinities." *Radical History Review* 119 (Spring 2014): 241–45. https://doi.org/10.1215/01636545-2402153.

Menon, Dilip M. 2017. "Was Mohandas Gandhi a Racist?" *Africa Is a Country* (blog). October 3. https://africasacountry.com/2017/03/was-mohandas-gandhi-a-racist.

Menon, Dilip M. 2018. "Thinking About the Global South." In *The Global South and Literature*, edited by Russell West-Pavlov, 34–44. Cambridge, UK: Cambridge University Press.

Menon, Pradeep. 2022. "The Data Mesh and the Hub-Spoke: A Macro Pattern for Scaling Analytics." *Medium*, March 14. https://rpradeepmenon.medium.com/the-data-mesh-and-the-hub-spoke-a-macro-pattern-for-scaling-analytics-9918fa67d8f2.

Metcalf, Thomas R. 1997. *Ideologies of the Raj.* Cambridge, UK: Cambridge University Press.

Mignolo, Walter. 2011. *The Darker Side of Western Modernity: Global Futures, Decolonial Options.* Durham, NC: Duke University Press.

Ministry of Finance. 2003. *Budget 2003–2004. Speech of Jaswant Singh, Minister of Finance and Company Affairs.* New Delhi, India. https://www.indiabudget.gov.in/doc/bspeech/bs200304.pdf.

Minn, Pierre. 2022. *Where They Need Me: Local Clinicians and the Workings of Global Health in Haiti.* Ithaca, NY: Cornell University Press.

Miscione, Gianluca. 2007. "Telemedicine in the Upper Amazon: Interplay with Local Health Care Practices." *MIS Quarterly* 31 (2): 403–25. https://doi.org/10.2307/25148797.

Mishra, Pankaj. 2013. "Which India Matters?" *New York Review of Books*, November 21. https://www.nybooks.com/articles/2013/11/21/which-india-matters.

Mishra, Saroj Kanta, Indra Pratap Singh, and Epu Daman Chand. 2012. "Current Status of Telemedicine Network in India and Future Perspective." *Proceedings of the Asia-Pacific Advanced Network* 32: 151–63.

Mitchell, Charlie. 2017. "Indian Healthcare Taps the African Market." *African Business*, May 29. https://african.business/2017/05/economy/indian-healthcare-taps -african-market.

Mitchell, Timothy. 2020. "Infrastructures Work on Time." *e-flux Architecture*, January. https://www.e-flux.com/architecture/new-silk-roads/312596/infrastructures -work-on-time.

Mkhwanazi, Nolwazi. 2016. "Medical Anthropology in Africa: The Trouble with a Single Story." *Medical Anthropology* 35 (2): 193–202. https://doi.org/10.1080/01459 740.2015.1100612.

Mkhwanazi, Nolwazi. 2020. "Of Dreams and Nightmares: Implementing Medical Male Circumcision in Eswatini (Swaziland)." *Africa* 90 (1): 132–47. https://doi.org /10.1017/S0001972019000974.

Ministry of External Affairs. 2012. *Connecting Hearts & Minds: India's PAN Africa Story*. Film by the Ministry of External Affairs, Government of India, 9 min., 28 sec. https://www.youtube.com/watch?v=eBUmdnab9io.

Modi, Renu. 2010. "The Role of India's Private Sector in the Health and Agricultural Sectors of Africa." In *The Rise of China & India in Africa*, edited by Fantu Cheru and Cyril Obi, 120–31. London: Zed.

Modi, Renu. 2011. "Offshore Healthcare Management: Medical Tourism Between Kenya, Tanzania and India." In *India in Africa. Changing Geographies of Power*, edited by Emma Mawdsley and Gerard McCann, 125–39. Oxford, UK: Pambazuka.

Mogaka, John J. O., Lucia Mupara, and Joyce M. Tsoka-Gwegweni. 2017. "Ethical Issues Associated with Medical Tourism in Africa." *Journal of Market Access & Health Policy* 5 (1): 1309770. https://doi.org/10.1080/20016689.2017.1309770.

Mol, Annemarie. 2002. *The Body Multiple. Ontology in Medical Practice*. Durham, NC: Duke University Press.

Mort, Maggie, Tracy Finch, and Carl May. 2009. "Making and Unmaking Telepatients: Identity and Governance in New Health Technologies." *Science Technology Human Values* 34 (1): 9–33. https://doi.org/10.1177/0162243907311274.

Moser, Ingunn, and John Law. 2006. "Fluids or Flows? Information and Qualculation in Medical Practice." *Information Technology & People* 19 (1): 55–73. https://doi .org/10.1108/09593840610649961.

Mullick, Rajeev. 2017. "King of Coins: This Guinness World Record Holder Has Over a Million of Them." *Hindustan Times*, May 8. https://www.hindustantimes.com /lucknow/meet-the-king-of-coins-who-has-gathered-a-million-of-them/story -0cpdrT1QMD1cR8BoHmZTtJ.html.

Mulot, Stéphanie, Sandrine Musso, and Juliette Sakoyan. 2011. "Médecines, mobilités et globalisation." *Anthropologie & Santé* 3. https://doi.org/10.4000/anthropolo giesante.718.

Munster, Anna. 2013. *An Aesthesia of Networks: Conjunctive Experience in Art and Technology*. Cambridge, MA: MIT Press.

Murphy, Michelle. 2017. *The Economization of Life*. Durham, NC: Duke University Press.

Nandy, Ashis. 1988. "Introduction: Science as a Reason of State." In *Science, Hegemony and Violence: A Requiem for Modernity*, edited by Ashis Nandy, 1–23. Tokyo: United Nations University.

Naraindas, Harish, and Cristiana Bastos. 2011. "Healing Holidays? Itinerant Patients, Therapeutic Locales and the Quest for Health." *Anthropology & Medicine* 18 (1): 1–6. https://doi.org/10.1080/13648470.2010.525871.

Narayana Hrudayalaya Healthcity. 2011. "Transforming Healthcare: Narayana Hrudayalaya Healthcity." Edited by Narayana Hrudayalaya Hospitals. Bangalore, India.

Ndong, Maguette. 2010. "Visite à la station terrienne de Gandoul—Moustapha Guirassy souligne l'importance des Tic." *Le Soleil*, March 10. http://www.osiris.sn/Visite-a -la-station-terrienne-de.html.

Nehru, Jawaharlal. 1947. "Pt. Jawaharlal Nehru's Speech: Asian Relations Conference 1947." *Tibet Sun*. Accessed October 18, 2024. https://www.tibetsun.com/news /1947/03/24/pt-jawaharlal-nehrus-speech-at-asian-relations-conference-1947.

Nehru, Jawaharlal. 1955. "Asia and Africa Awake. A Speech at the Concluding Session of the African Asian Conference at Bandung, Indonesia, April 24." In *Jawaharlal Nehru's Speeches, volume 3*. New Delhi: Ministry of Information and Broadcasting, Government of India, Publications Division.

Nehru, Jawaharlal. 1961. *India's Foreign Policy: Selected Speeches, September 1946–April 1961*. New Delhi: Publications Division, Ministry of Information and Broadcasting, Government of India.

Nehru, Jawaharlal. 1983. "An Address at the Indian Science Congress, Calcutta, 26 December 1937." In *Jawaharlal Nehru: An Anthology*, edited by Sarvepalli Gopal, 442. New Delhi, India: Oxford University Press.

Nehru, Jawaharlal. 2004. *The Discovery of India*. New Delhi, India: Penguin.

Neumark, Tom, and Ruth J. Prince. 2021. "Digital Health in East Africa: Innovation, Experimentation and the Market." *Global Policy* 12 (6): 65–74. https://doi.org /10.1111/1758-5899.12990.

Nguyen, Vinh-Kim. 2010. *The Republic of Therapy: Triage and Sovereignty in West Africa's Time of AIDS*. Durham, NC: Duke University Press.

Nilekani, Nandan. 2009. *Imagining India: The Idea of a Renewed Nation*. New Delhi, India: Penguin.

Nisbett, Nicholas. 2009. *Growing Up in the Knowledge Society: Living the IT Dream in Bangalore*. New Delhi, India: Routledge.

Olu, Olushayo, Derrick Muneene, Juliet Evelyn Bataringaya, Marie-Rosette Nahimana, Housseynou Ba, Yves Turgeon, Humphrey Cyprian Karamagi, and Delanyo Dovlo. 2019. "How Can Digital Health Technologies Contribute to Sustainable Attainment of Universal Health Coverage in Africa? A Perspective." *Frontiers in Public Health* 7: 341. https://doi.org/10.3389/fpubh.2019.00341.

Ormond, Meghann, and Heidi Kaspar. 2018. "South-South Medical Tourism." In *Routledge Handbook of South-South Relations*, edited by Elena Fiddian-Qasmiyeh and Patricia Daley, 397–405. Abingdon, UK: Routledge.

Oudshoorn, Nelly. 2012. "How Places Matter: Telecare Technologies and the Changing Spatial Dimension of Healthcare." *Social Studies of Science* 42 (1): 121–42. https:// doi.org/10.1177/0306312711431817.

Packard, Randall M. 2016. *A History of Global Health: Interventions into the Lives of Other Peoples*. Baltimore, MD: Johns Hopkins University Press.

Parks, Lisa. 2012. "Footprints of the Global South." *Handbook of Global Media Research*: 123–42. https://doi.org/10.1002/9781118255278.ch8.

Person, Donald A. 2000. "Pacific Island Health Care Project: Early Experiences with a Web-Based Consultation." *Pacific Health Dialog* 7 (2): 29–35. https://pubmed.ncbi .nlm.nih.gov/11588916.

Peters, John Durham. 1999. *Speaking into the Air: A History of the Idea of Communication*. Chicago: University of Chicago Press.

Peters, John Durham. 2015. *The Marvelous Clouds: Toward a Philosophy of Elemental Media*. Chicago: University of Chicago Press.

Peterson, Kristin. 2014. *Speculative Markets: Drug Circuits and Derivative Life in Nigeria*. Durham, NC: Duke University Press.

Peterson, Kristin, Morenike Oluwatoyin Folayan, Edward Chigwedere, and Evaristo Nthete. 2015. "Saying 'No' to PrEP research in Malawi: What Constitutes 'Failure' in Offshored HIV Prevention Research?" *Anthropology & Medicine* 22 (3): 278–94. https://doi.org/10.1080/13648470.2015.1081377.

Phạm, Quỳnh N., and Robbie Shilliam. 2016. "Reviving Bandung." In *Meanings of Bandung: Postcolonial Orders and Decolonial Visions*, edited by Quỳnh N Phạm and Robbie Shilliam, 3–19. London: Rowman & Littlefield.

Philip, Kavita. 2016. "Telling Histories of the Future: The Imaginaries of Indian Technoscience." *Identities* 23 (3): 276–93. https://doi.org/10.1080/1070289X.2015.1034129.

Pickering, Andrew. 1995. *The Mangle of Practice: Time, Agency, and Science.* Chicago: University of Chicago Press.

Pickles, Anthony J. 2023. "Comments on 'Expectations of the Gift.'" *Social Analysis* 67 (1): 92–96.

Pieters, C. M., J. N. Goswami, R. N. Clark, M. Annadurai, J. Boardman, B. Buratti, J-P. Combe, M. D. Dyar, R. Green, J. W. Head, C. Hibbitts, M. Hicks, P. Isaacson, R. Klima, G. Kramer, S. Kumar, E. Livo, S. Lundeen, E. Malaret, T. McCord, J. Mustard, J. Nettles, N. Petro, C. Runyon, M. Staid, J. Sunshine, L. A. Taylor, S. Tompkins, and P. Varanasi. 2009. "Character and Spatial Distribution of OH/H2O on the Surface of the Moon Seen by M^3 on Chandrayaan-1." *Science* 326 (5952): 568–72. https://doi.org/10.1126/science.1178658.

Pignarre, Philippe, and Isabelle Stengers. 2011. *Capitalist Sorcery: Breaking the Spell.* Translated by Andrew Goffey. New York: Palgrave Macmillan.

Planning Commission. 2002a. *India Vision 2020: The Report.* New Delhi, India: Academic Foundation, Government of India. https://py.gov.in/sites/default/files/indiavision2020.pdf.

Planning Commission. 2002b. *Tenth Five Year Plan 2002–07. Volume II: Sectoral Policies and Programmes.* New Delhi: Government of India.

Planning Commission. 2008. *Eleventh Five Year Plan (2007–2012). Volume I: Social Sector.* New Delhi: Government of India.

Pollock, Anne. 2019. *Synthesizing Hope: Matter, Knowledge, and Place in South African Drug Discovery.* Chicago: University of Chicago Press.

Pols, Jeannette. 2012. *Care at a Distance: On the Closeness of Technology.* Amsterdam: Amsterdam University Press.

Pols, Jeannette, and Ingunn Moser. 2009. "Cold Technologies Versus Warm Care? On Affective and Social Relations with and through Care Technologies." *ALTER, European Journal of Disability Research* 3: 159–78. https://doi.org/10.1016/j.alter.2009.01.003.

Porter, Michael E., and Thomas H. Lee. 2013. "The Strategy That Will Fix Health Care." *Harvard Business Review* https://hbr.org/2013/10/the-strategy-that-will-fix-health-care.

Povinelli, Elizabeth A. 2011. Routes/Worlds. *e-flux journal* 27. Accessed October 18, 2024. https://www.e-flux.com/journal/27/67991/routes-worlds/.

Prakash, Gyan. 1999. *Another Reason. Science and the Imagination of Modern India.* Princeton, NJ: Princeton University Press.

Prasad, Revati. 2018. "Ascendant India, Digital India: How Net Neutrality Advocates Defeated Facebook's Free Basics." *Media, Culture & Society* 40 (3): 415–31. https://doi.org/10.1177/0163443717736117.

Prashad, Vijay. 2002. *Everybody Was Kung Fu Fighting: Afro-Asian Connections and the Myth of Cultural Purity.* Boston: Beacon.

Prashad, Vijay. 2013. *The Poorer Nations: A Possible History of the Global South.* London: Verso.

Price, Gareth. 2004. *India's Aid Dynamics: From Recipient to Donor?* Asia Programme Working Paper, The Royal Institute of International Affairs, Chatham House, London. September. https://www.chathamhouse.org/sites/default/files/public/Research /Asia/wp200904.pdf.

Public Accounts Committee. 2005. "Twelfth Report (2004–2005): Allotment of Land to Private Hospitals and Dispensaries by Delhi Development Authority." Accessed June 14, 2024. https://eparlib.nic.in/bitstream/123456789/63261/1/14_Public _Accounts_12.pdf.

Puig de la Bellacasa, Maria. 2016. "Ecological Thinking, Material Spirituality, and the Poetics of Infrastructure." In *Boundary Objects and Beyond: Working with Leigh Star*, edited by Geoffrey C. Bowker, Stefan Timmermans, Adele E. Clarke, and Ellen Balka, 47–68. Cambridge, MA: MIT Press.

Qadeer, Imrana. 2000. "Health Care Systems in Transition. The Indian Experience." *Journal of Public Health Medicine* 22 (1): 25–32. https://doi.org/10.1093/pubmed /22.1.25.

Radha, Anu, and Sumit Osmand Shaw. 2011. *Connecting Hearts: India's Pan African e-Network*. Film, 8 min., 23 sec. Ministry of External Affairs, Government of India. https://www.youtube.com/watch?v=73LMVBnPacg.

Ramambazafy, Jeannot. 2010. "Madagascar Imailaka Télémédecine: le Futur est bien présent." *Madagate*, April 24, 2010. https://www.madagate.org/editorial/mad agate-video-et-affiche/1387-madagascar-imailaka-telemedecine-le-futur-est -bien-present.html.

Rao, Pavithra. 2017. "India's Medical Tourism Gets Africans' Attention." *Africa Renewal* 30 (3): 20–21. https://doi.org/10.18356/601440f0-en.

Rao, U. R. 1978. "An Overview of the 'Aryabhata' Project." *Proceedings of the Indian Academy of Sciences, Section C: Engineering Sciences* 1 (2): 117–33. https://doi .org/10.1007/BF02843538.

Rasquinha, David. 2016. "Healthcare in Africa, Built by India." In *Where Geopolitics Meets Business*, edited by Gateway House, 17–21. Mumbai, India: Gateway House: Indian Council on Global Relations. https://www.gatewayhouse.in/wp-content /uploads/2016/06/Where-Geopolitics-meets-Business.pdf.

Razgallah, Jamil. 2019. "Étude sur le vécu d'enfants cardiopathes et de leurs familles pris en charge par Terre des Hommes au Sénégal et en Suisse." Masters of Medicine, Faculté de biologie et de médecine, Université de Lausanne.

Redfield, Peter. 2000. *Space in the Tropics: From Convicts to Rockets in French Guiana*. Berkeley: University of California Press.

Redfield, Peter. 2013. *Life in Crisis: The Ethical Journey of Doctors without Borders*. Berkeley: University of California Press.

Roberts, Elizabeth F. S., and Nancy Scheper-Hughes. 2011. "Introduction: Medical Migra-tions." *Body & Society* 17 (2–3): 1–30. https://doi.org/10.1177/1357034X11400925.

Rockefeller Foundation. 2010. *From Silos to Systems: An Overview of eHealth's Transfor-mative Power*. New York: Rockefeller Foundation.

Rottenburg, Richard. 2009. *Far-Fetched Facts: A Parable of Development Aid*. Cam-bridge, MA: MIT Press.

Rottenburg, Richard, and Sally Engle Merry. 2015. "A World of Indicators: The Making of Governmental Knowledge through Quantification." In *A World of Indicators: The Making of Governmental Knowledge through Quantification*, edited by Rich-ard Rottenburg, Sally Engle Merry, Sung-Joon Park, and Johanna Mugler, 1–33. Cambridge, UK: Cambridge University Press.

Royall, Julia. 1998. "SatelLife: Linking Information and People: The Last Ten Centime-tres." *Development in Practice* 8 (1): 85–90.

Sagna, Olivier, Christophe Brun, and Steven Huter. 2013. *Historique de L'Internet au Sénégal (1989–2004)*. Eugene: University of Oregon Libraries.

Sahlins, Marshall. [2017] 1972. *Stone Age Economics*. New York: Routledge.

Sánchez-Criado, Tomás, Daniel López, Celia Roberts, and Miquel Domènech. 2014. "Installing Telecare, Installing Users: Felicity Conditions for the Instauration of Usership." *Science, Technology & Human Values* 39 (5): 694–719. https://doi.org /10.1177/0162243913517011.

Sarkar, Sreela. 2017. "Passionate Producers: Corporate Interventions in Expanding the Promise of the Information Society." *Communication, Culture & Critique* 10 (2): 241–60. https://doi.org/10.1111/cccr.12159.

Saunders, Barry F. 2008. *CT Suite: The Work of Diagnosis in the Age of Noninvasive Cutting*. Durham, NC: Duke University Press.

Sawadogo, N. Hélène, Hamidou Sanou, Jeremy A. Greene, and Vincent Duclos. 2021. "Promises and Perils of Mobile Health in Burkina Faso." *Lancet* 398 (10302): 738–39. https://doi.org/10.1016/S0140-6736(21)01001-1.

Scott, James C. 1985. *Weapons of the Weak: Everyday Forms of Peasant Resistance*. New Haven, CT: Yale University Press.

Scott, James C. 1998. *Seeing Like a State: How Certain Schemes to Improve the Human Condition Have Failed*. New Haven, CT: Yale University Press.

Scott Kruse, Clemens, Priyanka Karem, Kelli Shifflett, Lokesh Vegi, Karuna Ravi, and Matthew Brooks. 2018. "Evaluating Barriers to Adopting Telemedicine Worldwide: A Systematic Review." *Journal of Telemedicine and Telecare* 24 (1): 4–12. https://doi.org/10.1177/1357633X16674087.

Second Africa-India Forum Summit. 2011. *Africa-India Framework for Enhanced Cooperation*. Addis Ababa. http://www.au.int.

Sen, Gita. 2001. "Health Deteriorates." *The Hindu*, July 20. Accessed June 14, 2024. https://www.dawnnet.org/uploads/documents/ARTICLE_GITA_Health%20 Deteriorates_SRHR.pdf.

Senghor, Léopold Sédar. 1998. "Negritude and African Socialism." In *The African Philosophy Reader*, edited by P. H. Coetzee and A. P. J. Roux, 438–48. London: Routledge.

Sevilla-Buitrago, Alvaro. 2015. "Capitalist Formations of Enclosure: Space and the Extinction of the Commons." *Antipode* 47 (4): 999–1020. https://doi.org/10.1111/anti.12143.

Shah, Amrita. 2007. *Vikram Sarabhai: A Life*. Delhi, India: Penguin.

Shankar, Shobana. 2021. *An Uneasy Embrace: Africa, India and the Spectre of Race*. Oxford, UK: Oxford University Press.

Sharma, Mihir S. 2012. "Why Perry Anderson Is Wrong." *Business Standard*, November 1. https://www.business-standard.com/article/beyondbusiness/why-perry-ander son-is-wrong-112110100036_1.html.

Shaviro, Steven. 2003. *Connected, or, What It Means to Live in the Network Society. Electronic Mediations*. Minneapolis: University of Minnesota Press.

Sheehan, Michael. 2007. *The International Politics of Space*. London: Routledge.

Siddiqi, Asif. 2015. "Making Space for the Nation: Satellite Television, Indian Scientific Elites, and the Cold War." *Comparative Studies of South Asia, Africa & the Middle East* 35 (1): 35–49. https://doi.org/10.1215/1089201X-2876080.

Simondon, Gilbert. 1989. *L'individuation psychique et collective à la lumière des notions de forme, information, potentiel et métastabilité*. Paris: Aubier.

Simone, AbdouMaliq. 2018. "Inoperable Relations and Urban Change in the Global South." In *The Global South and Literature*, edited by Russell West-Pavlov, 123–33. Cambridge, UK: Cambridge University Press.

Singh, Bawa, Vijay Kumar Chattu, Jaspal Kaur, Rajni Mol, Priya Gauttam, and Balinder Singh. 2023. "COVID-19 and Global Distributive Justice: 'Health Diplomacy' of

India and South Africa for the TRIPS waiver." *Journal of Asian and African Studies* 58 (5): 747–65. https://doi.org/10.1177/00219096211069652.

Singh, Manmohan. 2004. *Prime Minister Dr. Manmohan Singh's Speech at the HT Leadership Initiative Conference, New Delhi—"India and the World: A Blueprint for Partnership and Growth."* New Delhi, India: Minister of External Affairs. https://www.mea.gov.in/Speeches-Statements.htm?dtl/3961/Prime.

Singh, Manmohan. 2011. "PM's Address at the Plenary Session of the 2nd Africa-India Forum Summit." Accessed September 30, 2024. https://pib.gov.in/newsite/PrintRelease.aspx?relid=72281.

Singh, Praney Kumar. 2010. "Indian Development Cooperation with Africa." In *The Rise of China & India in Africa: Challenges, Opportunities and Critical Interventions,* edited by Fantu Cheru and Cyril Obi, 77–93. New York: Zed.

Singh, Sinderpal. 2011. "From Delhi to Bandung: Nehru,'Indian-ness' and 'Pan-Asianness.'" *South Asia: Journal of South Asian Studies* 34 (1): 51–64. https://doi.org/10.1080/00856401.2011.549084.

Singh, Zorawar Daulet. 2019. "India's Civilisational Identity and the World Order." *Economic & Political Weekly* 54 (39): 10–12.

Sinha, Pranay Kumar. 2010. "Indian Development Cooperation with Africa." In *The Rise of China & India in Africa,* edited by Fantu Cheru and Cyril Obi, 77–93. London: Zed.

Six, Clemens. 2009. "The Rise of Postcolonial States as Donors: a Challenge to the Development Paradigm?" *Third World Quarterly* 30 (6): 1103–21. https://doi.org/10.1080/01436590903037366.

Sloterdijk, Peter. 2009. *Terror from the Air.* Translated by Amy Patton and Steve Corcoran. Los Angeles, CA: Semiotext(e).

Sloterdijk, Peter. 2012. "Nearness and *Da-sein*: The Spatiality of Being and Time." *Theory, Culture & Society* 29 (4/5): 36–42. https://doi.org/10.1177/0263276412448828.

Sloterdijk, Peter. 2013. *In the World Interior of Capital: Towards a Philosophical Theory of Globalization.* Translated by Wieland Hoban. Cambridge, UK: Polity.

Solomon, Harris. 2011. "Affective Journeys: The Emotional Structuring of Medical Tourism in India." *Anthropology and Medicine* 18 (1): 105–18. https://doi.org/10.1080/13648470.2010.525878.

Sprenger, Guido, Anthony J. Pickles, Ilana Gershon, Joel Robbins, Rebecca Bryant, and Marilyn Strathern. 2023. "Expectations of the Gift: Toward a Future-Oriented Taxonomy of Transactions: Article with Comments and Response." *Social Analysis* 67 (1): 70–124. https://doi.org/10.3167/sa.2023.670104. https://www.berghahnjournals.com/view/journals/social-analysis/67/1/sa670104.xml.

Srinivasan, Krishnan. 2019. "Values in Indian Foreign Policy: Lofty Ideals Give Way to Parochial Pragmatism." In *Values in Foreign Policy: Investigating Ideals and Interests,* edited by Krishnan Srinivasan, James Mayall, and Sanjay Pulipaka, 135–54. London: Rowman & Littlefield International.

Star, Susan Leigh. 1999. "The Ethnography of Infrastructure." *American Behavioral Scientist* 43 (3): 377–91. https://doi.org/10.1177/00027649921955326.

Star, Susan Leigh, and Karen Ruhleder. 1996. "Steps Toward an Ecology of Infrastructure: Design and Access for Large Information Spaces." *Information Systems Research* 7 (1): 111–34. https://doi.org/10.1287/isre.7.1.111.

Star, Susan Leigh, and Anselm Strauss. 1999. "Layers of Silence, Arenas of Voice: The Ecology of Visible and Invisible Work." *Computer Supported Cooperative Work* 8 (1): 9–30.

Starosielski, Nicole. 2015. *The Undersea Network.* Durham, NC: Duke University Press.

Stevenson, Lisa. 2014. *Life Beside Itself: Imagining Care in the Canadian Arctic*. Oakland: University of California Press.

Storeng, Katerini T., and Dominique P. Béhague. 2017. "'Guilty Until Proven Innocent': The Contested Use of Maternal Mortality Indicators in Global Health." *Critical Public Health* 27 (2): 163–76. https://doi.org/10.1080/09581596.2016.1259459.

Strathern, Marilyn. 1988. *The Gender of the Gift: Problems with Women and Problems with Society in Melanesia*. Berkeley: University of California Press.

Street, Alice. 2014. *Biomedicine in an Unstable Place: Infrastructure and Personhood in a Papua New Guinean Hospital*. London: Duke University Press.

Street, Alice, and Simon Coleman. 2012. "Introduction: Real and Imagined Spaces." *Space and Culture* 15 (1): 4–17. https://doi.org/10.1177/1206331211421852.

Subramaniam, Banu. 2019. *Holy Science: The Biopolitics of Hindu Nationalism*. Seattle: University of Washington Press.

Subramaniam, Banu. 2021. "Viral Fundamentals: Riding the Corona Waves in India." *Religion Compass* 15 (2): e12386. https://doi.org/10.1111/rec3.12386.

Sud, Nikita, and Diego Sánchez-Ancochea. 2022. "Southern Discomfort: Interrogating the Category of the Global South." *Development and Change* 53 (6): 1123–50. https://doi.org/10.1111/dech.12742.

Sundaram, Ravi. 2009. *Pirate Modernity: Delhi's Media Urbanism*. London: Routledge.

Sunder Rajan, Kaushik. 2006. *Biocapital. The Constitution of Postgenomic Life*. Durham, NC: Duke University Press.

Swinfen, R., and P. Swinfen. 2002. "Low-Cost Telemedicine in the Developing World." *Journal of Telemedicine and Telecare* 8 (suppl 2): 63–65. https://doi.org/10.1258/13576330260440899.

TallBear, Kim. 2011. "Why Interspecies Thinking Needs Indigenous Standpoints." *Cultural Anthropology*, Fieldsights, November 18. https://culanth.org/fieldsights/why-interspecies-thinking-needs-indigenous-standpoints.

The East African. 2015. "Rising Medical Bills Sending East African Patients Abroad." *The East African*, May 20. https://www.theeastafrican.co.ke/news/Rising-medical-bills-sending-East-African-patients-abroad/-/2558/2723450/-/139ke5gz/-/index.html.

The Hindu BusinessLine. 2021. "Vasudhaiva Kutumbakam Regards World as One Family: Modi at Quad Summit." *The Hindu BusinessLine*, March 12. https://www.thehindubusinessline.com/news/vasudhaiva-kutumbakam-regards-world-as-one-family-modi-at-quad-summit/article34054763.ece.

The Lancet. 1879. "Notes, Short Comments, and Answers to Correspondents." *The Lancet*, November 29: 819. https://doi.org/10.1016/S0140-6736(02)47536-8.

Thomas, George, and Suneeta Krishnan. 2010. "Effective Public-Private Partnership in Healthcare: Apollo as a Cautionary Tale." *Indian Journal of Medical Ethics* VII (1): 2–4. https://doi.org/10.20529/IJME.2010.001.

Thussu, Daya. 2013. *Communicating India's Soft Power: Buddha to Bollywood*. New York: Palgrave Macmillan.

Tomlinson, Mark, Mary Jane Rotheram-Borus, Leslie Swartz, and Alexander C. Tsai. 2013. "Scaling Up mHealth: Where Is the Evidence?" *PLoS Med* 10 (2): e1001382. https://doi.org/10.1371/journal.pmed.1001382.

Tompkins, Kyla Wazana. 2016. "On the Limits and Promise of New Materialist Philosophy." *Lateral: Journal of the Cultural Studies Association* 5 (1). https://doi.org/10.25158/L5.1.8.

Tsing, Anna. 2001. "Nature in the Making." In *New Directions in Anthropology and Environment: Intersections*, edited by Carole L. Crumley, 3–23. Lanham, MD: AltaMira Press.

Tsing, Anna. 2005. *Friction. An Ethnography of Global Connection*. Princeton, NJ: Princeton University Press.

Tsing, Anna. 2015. *The Mushroom at the End of the World: On the Possibility of Life in Capitalist Ruins*. Princeton, NJ: Princeton University Press.

Vaguet, Alain. 2009. "Introduction: Indian Health Landscapes under Globalization Treatment?" In *Indian Health Landscapes under Globalization*, edited by Alain Vaguet, 15–32. Delhi, India: CSH-Manohar.

Van Dijck, José. 2013. "Facebook and the Engineering of Connectivity: A Multi-Layered Approach to Social Media Platforms." *Convergence: The International Journal of Research into New Media Technologies* 19 (2): 141–55.

Van Eijk, Marieke. 2018. "The Anthropology of 'Boring' Things." *Medical Anthropology Quarterly Second Spear Blog Series* (blog). Last modified July 16, 2018. https://medanthroquarterly.org/second-spear/2018/07/the-anthropology-of-boring-things.

van Stam, Gertjan. 2022. "Conceptualization and Practices in Digital Health: Voices from Africa." *African Health Sciences* 22 (1): 664–72. https://doi.org/10.4314/ahs.v22i1.77.

Venkat, Bharat Jayram. 2021. *At the Limits of Cure*. Durham, NC: Duke University Press.

Venkatachalam, Meera, and Dan Banik. 2022. "Indian Exceptionalism and Normative Power in Africa." *African Arguments*, November 24. https://africanarguments.org/2022/11/indian-exceptionalism-and-normative-power-in-africa.

Vines, Alex. 2010. *India's Africa Engagement: Prospects for the 2011 India–Africa Forum*. Programme Paper: AFP 2010/01, Chatham House, London. December. https://www.chathamhouse.org/sites/default/files/public/Research/Africa/1210vines.pdf.

Visvanathan, Shiv. 2015. "APJ Abdul Kalam (1931–2015): Icon, Idol, Ascetic. . . ." *Open, the Magazine*, July 30. https://openthemagazine.com/essays/open-essay/apj-abdul-kalam-1931-2015-icon-idol-ascetic.

Vital Wave Consulting. 2012. *eTransform Africa: Health Sector Study. Sector Assessment and Opportunities for ICT*. Vital Wave Consulting. https://vitalwave.com/wp-content/uploads/2015/09/Complete-Report-Health.pdf.

Vitalis, Robert. 2013. "The Midnight Ride of Kwame Nkrumah and Other Fables of Bandung (Ban-doong)." *Humanity: An International Journal of Human Rights, Humanitarianism, and Development* 4 (2): 261–88. https://doi.org/10.1353/hum.2013.0018.

Viveiros de Castro, Eduardo. 2019. "On Models and Examples: Engineers and Bricoleurs in the Anthropocene." *Current Anthropology* 60 (S20): S296–S308. https://doi.org/10.1086/702787.

Wakhlu, Vimal. 2019. "How to Make the New NMC Bill More Effective and Acceptable: Vimal Wakhlu." *ET HealthWorld*, August 28. https://health.economictimes.indiatimes.com/news/policy/how-to-make-the-new-national-medical-commission-bill-more-effective-and-acceptable-to-all-the-stakeholders/70868339.

Wark, McKenzie. 2015. *Molecular Red: Theory for the Anthropocene*. New York: Verso.

Wark, McKenzie. 2016. "Friction." *Public Seminar* (blog). Last modified September 5, 2016. https://publicseminar.org/2016/09/friction/.

Warrier, Shobha. 2000. "Corporates Offer Hi-tech Health to Andhra's Villages." Rediff.com. Last modified April 14, 2000. http://www.rediff.com/business/2000/apr/14apollo.htm.

Weiner, Annette. 1992. *Inalienable Possessions: The Paradox of Keeping-While-Giving*. Berkeley: University of California Press.

WHO. 2004. *eHealth for Health-Care Delivery: Strategy 2004–2007*. Geneva: World Health Organization.

WHO. 2005a. *Connecting for Health: Global Vision. Local Insight.* Geneva: World Health Organization. https://iris.who.int/handle/10665/43385.

WHO. 2005b. *eHealth: Report by the Secretariat.* Geneva: World Health Organization. https://iris.who.int/handle/10665/20303.

WHO. 2005c. *Global eHealth Survey.* Geneva: World Health Organization.

WHO. 2010. *Telemedicine: Opportunities and Developments in Member States. Report on the Second Global Survey on eHealth.* Geneva: World Health Organization. https://iris.who.int/handle/10665/44497.

WHO. 2023. *Global Vaccine Market Report 2022: A Shared Understanding for Equitable Access to Vaccines.* Geneva: World Health Organization. https://www.who.int/publications/i/item/9789240062726.

Wilson, K., B. Gertz, B. Arenth, and N. Salisbury. 2014. *The Journey to Scale: Moving Together Past Digital Health Pilots.* Seattle, WA: PATH.

Wool, Zoe H., and Julie Livingston. 2017. "Collateral Afterworlds: An Introduction." *Social Text* 35, no. 1 (130): 1–15. https://doi.org/10.1215/01642472-3727960.

Woolgar, Steve, and Javier Lezaun. 2013. "The Wrong Bin Bag: A Turn to Ontology in Science and Technology Studies?" *Social Studies of Science* 43 (3): 321–40. https://doi.org/10.1177/0306312713488820.

Wynter, Sylvia. 1989. "Beyond the Word of Man: Glissant and the New Discourse of the Antilles." *World Literature Today* 63 (4): 637–48. https://doi.org/10.2307/40145557.

Xue, Yajiong, Huigang Liang, Victor Mbarika, Richard Hauser, Paul Schwager, and Mequanint Kassa Getahun. 2015. "Investigating the Resistance to Telemedicine in Ethiopia." *International Journal of Medical Informatics* 84 (8): 537–47. https://doi.org/10.1016/j.ijmedinf.2015.04.005.

Yan, Yunxiang. 2023. "Gifts." In *The Open Encyclopedia of Anthropology,* edited by Felix Stein. http://doi.org/10.29164/20gifts.

Yong, Dongeun, Mark A. Toleman, Christian G. Giske, Hyun S. Cho, Kristina Sundman, Kyungwon Lee, and Timothy R. Walsh. 2009. "Characterization of a New Metallo-β-lactamase Gene, bla NDM-1, and a Novel Erythromycin Esterase Gene Carried on a Unique Genetic Structure in Klebsiella Pneumoniae Sequence Type 14 from India." *Antimicrobial Agents and Chemotherapy* 53 (12): 5046–54. https://doi.org/10.1128/AAC.00774-09.

Index

action at a distance, 115, 174nn39–41. *See also* distance, the production of
actor-network theory, 71, 152n11
Addis Ababa, 11, 17–18, 32, 51, 82, 86, 137
Addis Ababa Declaration, 157–58n30
Adibe, Jideofor, 148
affect. *See* PAN, affect and affective investment
Africa-India Framework for Enhanced Cooperation, 109
African Union (AU), 137, 145, 146, 150, 151n3,157n26
African Union Commission (AUC), 11, 57, 58, 127, 132, 145, 152n15, 163n27
Alcatel Submarine Networks, 61. *See also* undersea cables
All India Institute of Medical Sciences (AIIMS, New Delhi), 17, 51, 93, 109, 159n37
Ambedkar, B. R. (politician), 101
Ambedkar, Dr. (PAN doctor), 51, 52, 53, 54, 162n11
Apollo Hospital (Chennai), 1, 6, 17, 45, 51, 52, 67–68, 73, 79, 84, 98, 122
Apollo Hospitals (company), 13, 17, 37, 82–85, 90, 98, 99, 105, 109, 126, 161n8, 166n16
Apollo Tele Health Services, 91
Apollo Telemedicine Networking Foundation (ATNF) 1, 37, 68, 73, 74
history of, 17, 38, 99, 159n43
See also corporate hospitals, in India; telemedicine in India
archipelago of care and expertise, 7–8, 78–79, 82, 86, 152n18. *See also* enclosure and insulation; global capitalism
ATLANTIS-2, 5, 61–63, 72, 163n34, 164n36. *See also* undersea cables

Bandung Conference, 3, 9, 19, 25–28, 36, 43, 110, 143, 155n10, 157n21, 173n25. *See also* South-South cooperation
Bangalore, 37, 85, 87, 99, 105, 145, 166n13
Barad, Karen, 71, 152n11
Berlant, Lauren, 174n33
Bill and Melinda Gates Foundation, 8

Bharatiya Janata Party (BJP), 31, 171n7, 172n23
Bharti Airtel, 60–61, 163n32
Black Lion Hospital (Addis Ababa), 51, 86, 87, 96, 137
Bosaso General Hospital (Bosaso), 6, 51, 74, 75
Bose, Dr., 91
Bowker, Geoffrey, 174n36
Boyer, Dominic, 107

capitalist dreams and dream-making, in India, 3, 12, 14, 21, 98, 99, 100, 102–3, 140. *See also* Kalam, Abdul; PAN, affect and affective investment; PAN, speculative project
CARE hospital (Hyderabad), 137
Césaire, Aimé, 143
Chakrabarty, Dipesh, 9, 27, 175n50
Chamayou, Grégoire, 164n45
Chatterjee, Partha, 153n20
Chen, Kuan-Hsing, 32
Chennai. *See* Apollo Hospital (Chennai)
CHNU Fann, 4, 5, 17, 18, 44–48, 49, 50, 51, 52, 54, 55, 56, 57, 63–64, 66, 68–69, 80, 81, 82, 85, 87, 91, 92, 93, 96, 118, 123, 128, 129, 132, 138, 149, 150
Centre Cardio-pédiatrique Cuomo, 150
Department of Cardiology, 44–45, 48–49, 52–53
Department of Neurology, 50
Department of Thoracic and Cardiovascular Surgery (DTCS), 45, 53–56, 162n15
history of pediatric surgery, 4, 49, 51, 56
other telemedicine projects, 47, 180n51
as regional hub, 47, 56
as transit space, 54
China. *See* India-Africa relations: comparison/competition with China
Chopra, Dr., 45
Clinical space (in telemedicine), 21, 90, 97
clinic as material and technical space, 5, 18, 46, 57, 70, 78 (*see also* PAN, design and implementation)
clinical work (*see* PAN, telemedicine)

www.ingramcontent.com/pod-product-compliance
Lightning Source LLC
Chambersburg PA
CBHW030322270326
41926CB00010B/1465